SOMATIC EXERCISE
FOR BEGINNERS

Regenerate your body and mind from stress, anxiety, and emotional tension. Learn to boost your energy and physical strength in under 15 minutes a day.

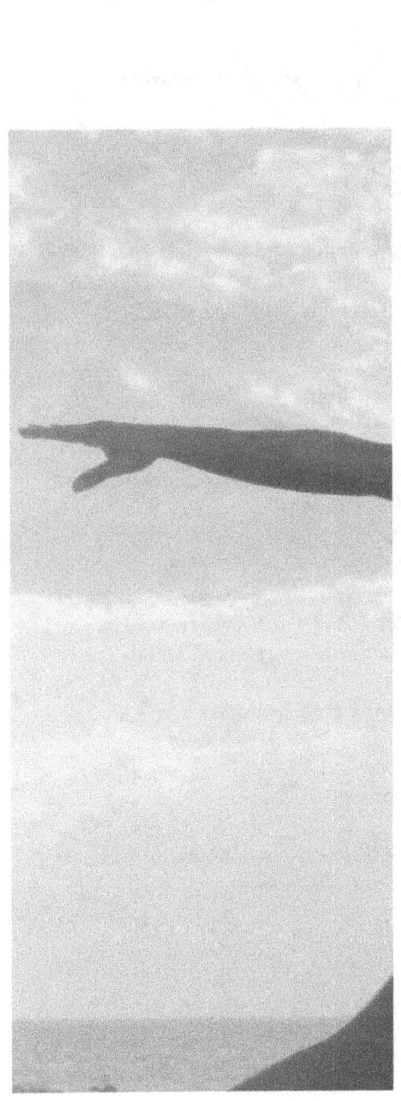

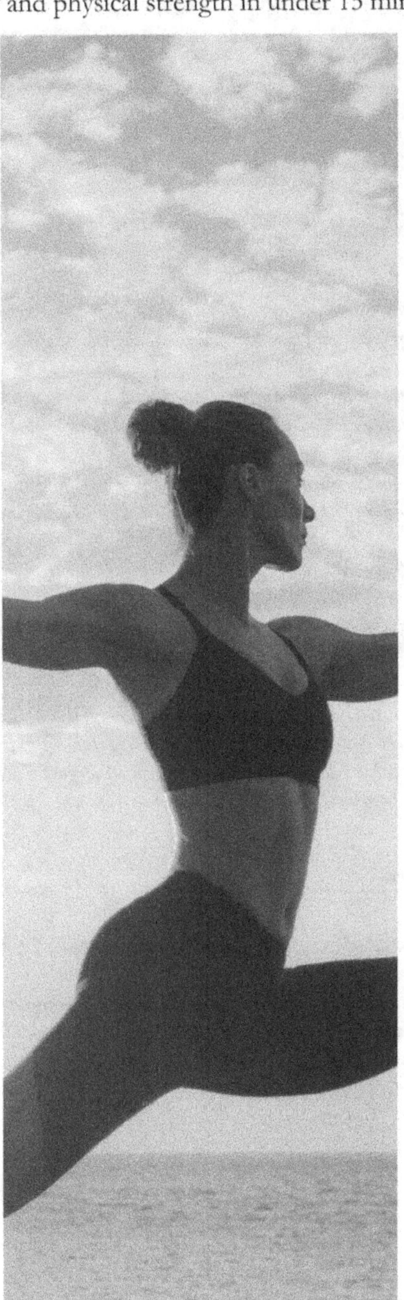

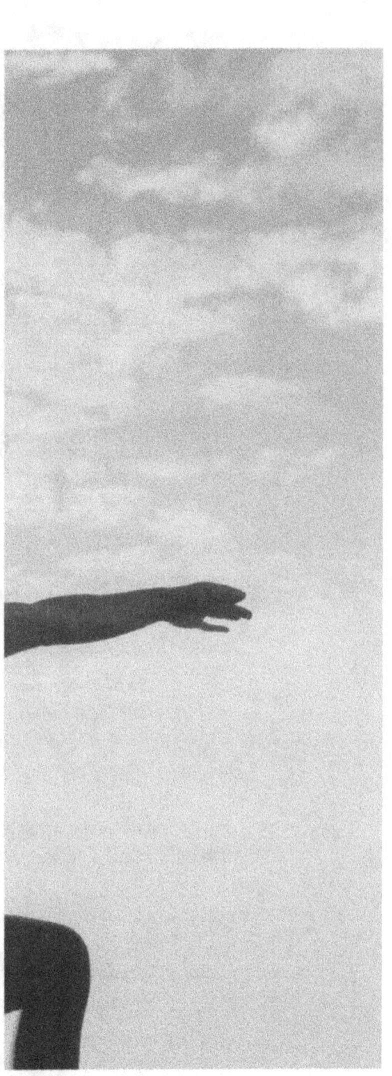

By: Dr. Shara Puenta

Table of Contents

History and Definition

Somatic yoga is a holistic practice that integrates the principles of somatics with traditional yoga techniques. The term "somatics" originates from the Greek word "soma," meaning "body," and focuses on the internal experience of the body rather than its external appearance. This practice emerged in the mid-20th century through the work of pioneers like Thomas Hanna, who coined the term "somatics" to describe a field of study that emphasizes internal physical perception and experience. Somatic yoga blends these principles with traditional yoga, creating a practice that prioritizes gentle, mindful movement and heightened body awareness. It aims to release chronic tension, improve mobility, and foster a deeper connection between the mind and body.

How Somatic Yoga Differs from Traditional Yoga

Somatic yoga stands out from traditional yoga through its unique focus on the internal experience of movement and the mind-body connection. While traditional yoga often emphasizes achieving specific postures and maintaining external alignment, somatic yoga invites practitioners to turn their attention inward. The goal is not to perfect the pose but to explore how each movement feels, cultivating a deeper awareness of the body's sensations and responses. This approach encourages a more personalized practice, where each individual can move in a way that feels right for their own body.

Internal Experience Over External Form

In traditional yoga, especially styles like Hatha Yoga, the emphasis is often on achieving and holding specific postures (asanas) with proper external alignment. Somatic yoga, on the other hand, prioritizes the internal experience of movement. Practitioners focus on how each movement feels from the inside, using this awareness to release tension and improve movement patterns. This shift from external form to internal experience fosters a more intuitive and personalized practice.

Reprogramming the Brain-to-Muscle Connection

One of the main differences between traditional Hatha Yoga and Gentle Somatic Yoga (GSY) is the focus on reprogramming and strengthening the brain-to-muscle connection rather than stretching muscles. This is achieved through a technique called pandiculation, which involves contracting a muscle group and then slowly releasing the contraction while maintaining awareness of the movement. Pandiculation helps reset the nervous system and restore natural movement patterns, leading to greater ease and freedom of movement.

Accessibility and Adaptability

Somatic yoga is designed to be inclusive and adaptable, making it accessible to individuals of all ages and fitness levels. The movements are gentle and can be modified to suit various physical conditions. This contrasts with some traditional yoga practices that may require a higher level of physical fitness and flexibility. Somatic yoga's adaptability ensures that everyone can participate and benefit from the practice, regardless of their starting point.

Emphasis on Relaxation and Release

Traditional yoga can sometimes be physically demanding, focusing on building strength and flexibility through challenging postures. In contrast, somatic yoga emphasizes relaxation and the release of tension. The practice includes a significant amount of time spent in restorative poses and gentle stretches, which help calm the nervous system and promote deep relaxation. This focus on relaxation is particularly beneficial for individuals dealing with chronic stress and tension.

Integration of Somatic Principles

Somatic yoga incorporates principles from somatic education, such as sensory awareness, proprioception, and neuro-muscular re-education. These principles help practitioners develop a deeper understanding of their body's movement patterns and make conscious adjustments to improve their overall function. This integration adds a layer of depth to the practice, enhancing its therapeutic benefits and making it a valuable tool for physical and mental health.

Embracing the Mind-Body Connection

At the heart of somatic yoga is the profound connection between the mind and body. This practice deeply integrates meditation, emphasizing mindfulness in every movement. Unlike some traditional yoga practices where meditation and movement are separate, in somatic yoga, they are seamlessly intertwined. This integration transforms each movement into a form of moving meditation, where practitioners remain fully present and aware of their body's sensations.

Mindful Movement

Mindful movement is a core aspect of somatic yoga. Practitioners are encouraged to perform each movement with full attention, cultivating a state of meditative focus. This mindful approach helps enhance the connection between the mind and body, promoting greater harmony and balance. By staying present and aware during practice, individuals can experience a deeper sense of self-awareness and inner peace.

Breath Awareness

Breath awareness is another crucial element in somatic yoga. Practitioners learn to synchronize their breath with their movements, using deep, conscious breathing to enhance relaxation and focus. This breath awareness helps anchor the mind in the present moment, fostering a sense of calm and clarity. By paying close attention to the breath, practitioners can deepen their connection to their body and enhance the overall effectiveness of their practice.

Sensory Exploration

Somatic yoga encourages practitioners to explore their body's sensations with curiosity and openness, without judgment. This sensory exploration is a form of meditation that enhances self-awareness and promotes healing. By tuning into the subtleties of movement and sensation, individuals can develop a deeper understanding of their body's needs and responses.

Stress Reduction

The meditative aspects of somatic yoga are particularly effective for stress reduction. By focusing on gentle, mindful movement and deep breathing, practitioners can activate the body's relaxation response, reducing the impact of stress on both the mind and body. This practice promotes a sense of inner peace and well-being, helping individuals navigate the challenges of daily life with greater ease and resilience.

Somatic Awareness

Somatic awareness is the foundational principle of somatic yoga, emphasizing the importance of being fully present in your body and attuned to its sensations. It involves a heightened state of body consciousness, where you actively listen to and feel your body from the inside. This internal focus helps you recognize patterns of tension, movement habits, and areas that need attention or release.

By developing somatic awareness, you learn to move with more intention and understanding. This practice encourages you to pay attention to how your body feels during each movement, rather than simply aiming for an external appearance. Over time, this awareness can lead to improved posture, reduced pain, and a greater sense of ease and fluidity in your movements.

The Role of Breath in Somatic Practices

Breath plays a crucial role in somatic yoga, serving as a bridge between the mind and body. It helps regulate the nervous system, promotes relaxation, and enhances the effectiveness of movements. Understanding the timing and aspects of breath in somatic practices is essential for reaping the full benefits.

Breath Awareness

Breath awareness is the practice of focusing on your breathing patterns. In somatic yoga, you start by simply observing your breath without trying to change it. Notice the rhythm, depth, and quality of your breaths. This initial awareness sets the stage for more intentional breathing practices.

Deep Breathing

Deep breathing involves taking slow, full breaths that expand the diaphragm and fill the lungs completely. This type of breathing helps activate the parasympathetic nervous system, promoting relaxation and reducing stress. In somatic yoga, deep breathing is often synchronized with movements to enhance the mind-body connection.

Timing of Breathing

The timing of your breath in somatic yoga is synchronized with your movements. Here are some general guidelines:

- **Inhalation**: Inhale during movements that open or expand the body, such as reaching upward or arching the back. This helps to energize and create space within the body.
- **Exhalation**: Exhale during movements that close or contract the body, such as folding forward or curling inward. This aids in relaxation and release of tension.
- **Natural Pause**: Allow for a natural pause between inhalation and exhalation. This brief moment of stillness can enhance the sense of calm and mindfulness.

Breath and Movement Synchronization

Synchronizing breath with movement involves coordinating each inhale and exhale with specific actions. For example, in a simple forward fold, you might inhale to lengthen the spine and exhale to fold forward, allowing the breath to guide and deepen the movement. This synchronization creates a seamless flow, making each movement more intentional and mindful.

Sensitivity and mindfulness are integral components of somatic yoga. They involve cultivating a deep awareness of your body's sensations and responses, as well as maintaining a present-focused, non-judgmental attitude.

Cultivating Sensitivity

Cultivating sensitivity means becoming more attuned to the subtle signals your body sends. This includes noticing areas of tension, discomfort, or ease and responding to these sensations with gentle, mindful movements. By regularly practicing somatic yoga, you develop a refined sense of body awareness that can help prevent injury and promote overall well-being.

Practicing Mindfulness

Mindfulness in somatic yoga involves staying fully present in each moment, paying attention to your body, breath, and mind without judgment. This practice encourages you to let go of distractions and focus entirely on the experience of movement and sensation.

Simple Meditation Practice for Relief

Here's a simple meditation practice to cultivate sensitivity and mindfulness, providing relief from stress and tension:

Body Scan Meditation

1. **Find a Comfortable Position**: Sit or lie down in a comfortable position. Close your eyes and take a few deep breaths to settle in.

2. **Focus on Your Breath**: Begin by bringing your attention to your breath. Notice the rise and fall of your chest or abdomen with each inhale and exhale.

3. **Scan Your Body**: Start at the top of your head and slowly move your attention down through your body. As you scan each area, notice any sensations, tension, or discomfort. Spend a few moments on each part, simply observing without trying to change anything.

4. **Release Tension**: When you encounter areas of tension, imagine sending your breath to that spot. Inhale deeply, and as you exhale, visualize the tension melting away. Continue this process as you move down through your body.

5. **Stay Present**: Throughout the body scan, maintain a non-judgmental attitude. If your mind wanders, gently bring it back to the present moment and your breath.

6. **Finish with Deep Breaths**: Once you have scanned your entire body, take a few more deep breaths. Notice how your body feels now compared to when you started.

7. **Gently Transition**: When you're ready, slowly open your eyes and take a moment to reorient yourself before moving on with your day.

How to Stay Motivated

Staying motivated in your somatic yoga practice is essential for achieving lasting benefits. Consistency is the key to developing deeper body awareness, relieving stress, and fostering overall well-being. Establishing a routine tailored to your needs and goals can make all the difference in maintaining your motivation and ensuring long-term success.

The Importance of Consistency

Consistency in somatic yoga practice builds a strong foundation for physical and mental health. Regular practice helps to reinforce the mind-body connection, making it easier to access relaxation and mindfulness in daily life. By practicing consistently, you create positive habits that become second nature, reducing the effort needed to maintain your routine.

Establishing a Routine

Creating a structured routine is crucial for staying motivated, especially for those with busy lifestyles. A well-defined routine provides a sense of stability and predictability, making it easier to integrate somatic yoga into your daily life. Here's a suggested daily routine focused on stress relief and mindfulness:

Personalizing Your Practice

Tailor your routine to suit your personal preferences and lifestyle. If mornings are too hectic, consider practicing in the evening when you have more time to unwind. The key is to find a schedule that you can consistently maintain and that feels natural to you.

Tips to Stay Motivated

Set Clear Goals

Having clear, achievable goals can provide direction and purpose for your practice. Set both short-term and long-term goals. Short-term goals might include practicing three times a week or mastering a specific movement, while long-term goals could focus on overall stress reduction or improved body awareness. Regularly review and adjust your goals to keep them relevant and challenging.

Track Your Progress

Keeping a journal or using a tracking app can help you monitor your progress and stay motivated. Record your practice sessions, note any changes in your physical or mental state, and celebrate your achievements. Seeing tangible progress can boost your motivation and reinforce the benefits of your practice.

Create a Supportive Environment

Your practice environment plays a significant role in maintaining motivation. Designate a quiet, comfortable space for your somatic yoga practice. Ensure it's free from distractions and equipped with any props you might need, such as a yoga mat, blankets, or pillows. A serene environment can enhance your focus and make your practice more enjoyable.

Connect with a Community

Joining a community of like-minded individuals can provide support, encouragement, and accountability. Participate in local or online somatic yoga classes, workshops, or forums. Engaging with others who share your interests can provide new insights, keep you inspired, and help you stay committed to your practice.

Celebrate Small Wins

Acknowledge and celebrate your progress, no matter how small. Recognizing your achievements can boost your confidence and motivation. Treat yourself to something special when you reach a milestone, such as a new yoga prop, a relaxing bath, or a favorite healthy snack.

Mix It Up

Variety can keep your practice interesting and prevent burnout. Incorporate different somatic exercises, try new meditation techniques, or explore other aspects of somatic awareness. Mixing up your routine can keep you engaged and excited about your practice.

Practice Self-Compassion

Be kind to yourself and understand that motivation can fluctuate. There will be days when it's harder to practice, and that's okay. Instead of being critical, practice self-compassion. Recognize that taking even a few minutes for mindful breathing or gentle movement is a step in the right direction.

Remind Yourself of the Benefits

Regularly remind yourself of the benefits you experience from your practice. Reflect on how somatic yoga has improved your physical and mental well-being, reduced your stress, or enhanced your body awareness. Keeping these benefits in mind can reinforce your motivation and commitment.

Common Sources of Pain and Tension

Many individuals, especially those with busy and demanding lifestyles, often experience various forms of pain and tension. Understanding the common sources of these issues can help in addressing them effectively through somatic yoga. Here are some of the most prevalent sources of pain and tension:

1. Neck and Shoulder Tension

- **Causes**: Prolonged sitting, poor posture, stress, and repetitive movements can lead to tightness and discomfort in the neck and shoulders.
- **Symptoms**: Stiffness, reduced range of motion, headaches, and chronic tension.

2. Lower Back Pain

- **Causes**: Sedentary lifestyle, poor posture, improper lifting techniques, and weak core muscles.
- **Symptoms**: Sharp or dull pain in the lower back, muscle spasms, and difficulty standing up straight.

3. Hip and Pelvic Discomfort

- **Causes**: Prolonged sitting, imbalanced muscle use, and lack of flexibility.
- **Symptoms**: Pain in the hips, lower back, and groin area, along with reduced mobility.

4. Joint Pain

- **Causes**: Aging, arthritis, repetitive strain injuries, and lack of movement.
- **Symptoms**: Swelling, stiffness, and pain in the joints, particularly in the knees, wrists, and fingers.

5. Muscle Tension

- **Causes**: Stress, overuse, dehydration, and poor ergonomics.
- **Symptoms**: Tightness, knots, and soreness in various muscle groups.

6. Chronic Stress and Anxiety

- **Causes**: Work pressure, personal issues, lack of relaxation, and mental health conditions.
- **Symptoms**: Generalized body tension, headaches, digestive issues, and fatigue.

In the following chapters, this book provides a series of detailed exercises specifically designed to address common sources of pain and tension. Each exercise is explained with clear instructions, focusing on particular body positions and movements that target pain points effectively.

Pregnancy is a unique journey, one filled with excitement, wonder, and a fair share of challenges. It's a time when your body and mind undergo incredible transformations as you prepare to welcome new life. Amidst the whirlwind of changes, yoga can become a sanctuary—a gentle, supportive practice that helps you glide through these months with grace and ease. Let's explore how yoga can make this beautiful journey smoother, more comfortable, and deeply fulfilling.

Embracing the Changes with Mobility

Imagine your body as a flowing river, constantly adapting to the new life growing within. Some days, you might feel like a graceful swan, while other days, you might feel more like a clumsy duckling. Yoga can be your ally in maintaining mobility and grace.

As your belly grows, simple movements can become tricky. Yoga helps keep your body flexible and strong, especially in the hips, back, and legs. Think of poses like Cat-Cow, which gently stretches your spine, or Child's Pose, which offers a soothing stretch for your back. These poses make daily movements easier and help you feel more at home in your changing body.

Balance can also be a challenge as your center of gravity shifts. Poses like Tree Pose or Warrior II can help you find your footing, literally and figuratively, giving you the stability you need to move with confidence.

Easing the Aches and Pains

Pregnancy often brings its share of aches and pains, particularly in the lower back, hips, and legs. Yoga can be a lifesaver here, offering gentle, effective relief.

Back pain, for instance, is a common companion during pregnancy. Gentle movements like Cat-Cow and Pelvic Tilts can ease the pressure on your spine, making everything from sitting to sleeping more comfortable.

Hip pain can also be a real nuisance. Poses like Pigeon Pose or Bound Angle Pose open up the hips, relieving tension and discomfort. And if you're dealing with sciatic pain—a sharp, shooting pain that runs from your lower back down your leg—yoga can help ease this too, with stretches that gently release the pressure on your sciatic nerve.

Finding Calm in the Chaos

Beyond the physical benefits, yoga is a wonderful tool for nurturing your mental and spiritual health during pregnancy. The emotional rollercoaster of these months can be intense, but yoga offers a way to find calm and clarity amidst the chaos.

Deep breathing exercises and meditation can be incredibly soothing, helping to reduce stress and anxiety. When you focus on your breath, you activate your parasympathetic nervous system, which promotes relaxation and well-being. It's like hitting the pause button on your busy mind, giving you a moment of peace.

Yoga also fosters emotional stability. By encouraging mindfulness, it helps you stay present and connected to your emotions, allowing you to navigate the highs and lows with greater ease. And then there's the spiritual aspect. Pregnancy is a deeply spiritual time, and yoga can enhance this connection. Through practices like guided meditation, gentle asanas, and even chanting, you can cultivate a deeper bond with your baby and a profound sense of inner peace.

A Heartwarming Story

Take the story of Sarah, for example. She was overwhelmed with the physical changes and emotional stresses of pregnancy. She found her refuge in prenatal yoga classes. The gentle movements eased her back pain, and the breathing exercises helped her manage anxiety. Sarah often spoke of how yoga became her anchor, allowing her to connect deeply with her baby and herself. Her yoga practice became a cherished time of day where she could focus on her well-being, fostering a sense of calm and readiness for the journey ahead.

Dandasana (Staff Pose)

Dandasana, or Staff Pose, is a foundational seated posture that helps improve posture and alignment, setting the tone for the rest of your yoga practice. Although it might seem simple, this pose embodies many elements essential to your overall practice: activated back and shoulders, strong posture, and engagement from the crown of your head to your feet. Dandasana aligns your body similarly to Tadasana (Mountain Pose) and serves as a vital reference for maintaining proper alignment. Imagining your spine as a vertical staff firmly rooted in the Earth can help enhance your awareness and support throughout your yoga journey.

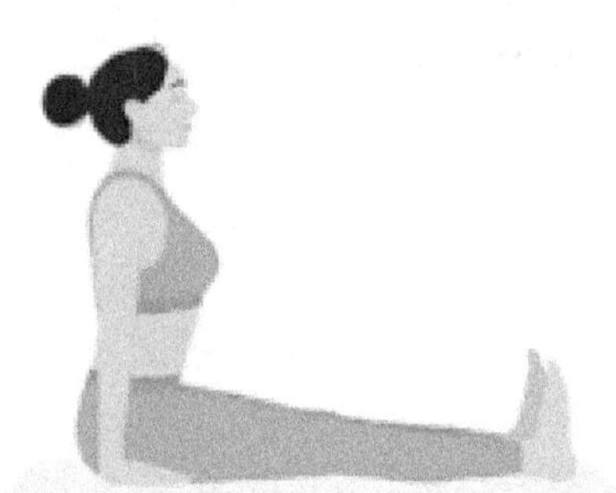

Starting Position
- Get into a sitting position on the floor, legs spread forward.
- Sit with your back straight and your legs together, touching your big toes and keeping a small space between your heels.

Position Your Hands
- Place your hands alongside your hips and straighten your arms.
- Put your hands on books, blocks, or folded blankets to make the ground closer if they can't reach the mat.

Engage Your Legs and Feet
- Flex your ankles and draw your toes back towards you.
- Press forward with your big toe mounds.
- Rotate your inner thighs inward and press them down into the mat.

Align Your Spine
- Spread your collarbones wide and pull your sternum away from your belly button.
- While releasing tension in your front ribs, bring the tips of your upper arms back.

Maintain Proper Alignment
- Ensure your sacrum and shoulder blades are touching the wall (if using a wall for support) but not your lower back or the back of your head.
- Imagine your spine as a vertical staff firmly rooted in the Earth.

Breathe and Hold
- Inhale deeply to lengthen your spine.
- Exhale and maintain the engagement in your legs, core, and back.
- Hold the pose for several breaths, focusing on your alignment and steady breathing.

- To exit the pose, release your arms and shake out your legs.

Key Points
- Keep your spine long and straight, avoiding rounding your back.
- Flex your feet and press your thighs down into the mat.
- Ensure your sacrum and shoulder blades are aligned and your shoulders are drawn back.

Variation:

Staff Pose Against a Wall

Starting Position
- Sit on the floor with your legs stretched out in front of you, back against a wall.
- Sit on one or more folded blankets if needed to elevate your hips and maintain a straight spine.

Position Your Legs
- Touch your big toes together and keep a small space between your heels.
- Flex your ankles, drawing your toes back towards you.
- Bring your inner thighs in toward your body and press them into the mat while your big toes push forward.

Align Your Back
- Ensure your sacrum and shoulder blades are touching the wall, but your lower back and the back of your head are not.
- Extend your collarbones wide and pull your sternum away from your belly button.

Position Your Hands
- Place your hands alongside your hips and straighten your arms.
- To make room on the mat, prop your hands up on books, blocks, or folded blankets.

Engage and Lengthen
- While releasing tension in your front ribs, bring the tips of your upper arms back. Imagine your spine as a vertical staff firmly rooted in the Earth.

Breathe and Hold
- Inhale deeply to lengthen your spine.
- Exhale and maintain the engagement in your legs, core, and back.
- Hold the pose for several breaths, focusing on your alignment and steady breathing.

By using a wall for support, this variation of Dandasana helps you maintain proper alignment and provides additional stability, making it easier to focus on engaging the necessary muscles and maintaining a straight spine.

Paschimottanasana, or Seated Forward Bend, is an ancient Hatha yoga posture that stretches your back deeply, beginning at the base of your skull and working its way up the body. This pose is especially beneficial for runners with tight hamstrings and is known for its calming effects, helping to relieve stress and improve mood. Additionally, Seated Forward Bend stretches the hamstrings, shoulders, and lower back, lengthens the spine, invigorates the nervous system, and stimulates the abdominal organs, improving digestion. It can also ease symptoms of menstruation and menopause while relieving stress, anxiety, and mild depression.

Starting Position
- Position yourself on the floor, legs stretched straight.
- Put your hands on the mat beside your hips, press down to flex your feet and lift your torso into Dandasana.

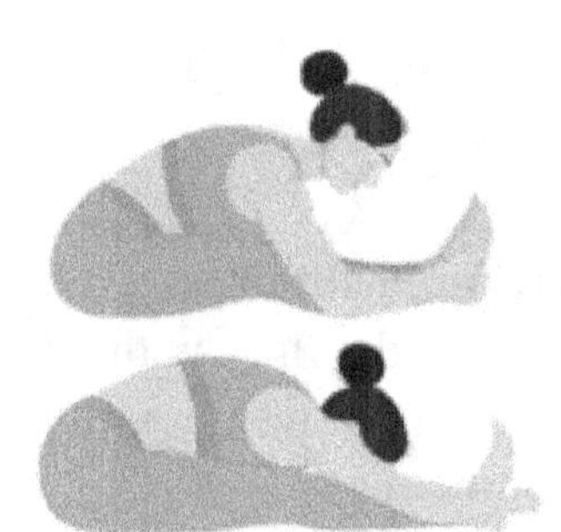

Hinge Forward
- Inhale and lengthen your spine, grounding down through your sitting bones.
- Exhale and tilt forward at your hips, folding over your thighs with a straight spine.

Reach Forward
- Place your arms out to the sides and reach them up over your head, all the way to the sky.
- Inhale to draw your spine up long.
- Exhale and continue to hinge forward, imagining your pelvis as a bowl of water tipping forward.

Engage and Stretch
- On each inhale, lift and lengthen your torso slightly.
- On each exhale, deepen the forward bend, aiming to bring your belly toward your thighs rather than your nose to your knees.

Hold the Pose
- Take hold of your ankles and shins, or use a strap around your feet if needed.
- Keep your feet flexed and your neck as a natural extension of your spine.
- Hold the pose for 8-10 breaths, breathing deeply and evenly.

Release the Pose
- Inhale and gently lift your torso back up, coming out of the forward bend.
- Exhale and return to Dandasana.

Key Points
- As you bend forward, make sure to maintain a long and straight spine.
- Keep your feet flexed throughout the pose to enhance the stretch in your hamstrings.
- Use your inhales to lengthen the spine and your exhales to deepen the forward bend.

Variation:

Chair Seated Forward Bend

Starting Position
- Sit near the front edge of your chair.
- Separate your feet so your thighs are 90 degrees apart and your knees are directly over your ankles.
- Point your feet in the same direction as your thighbones and place your hands on your knees.

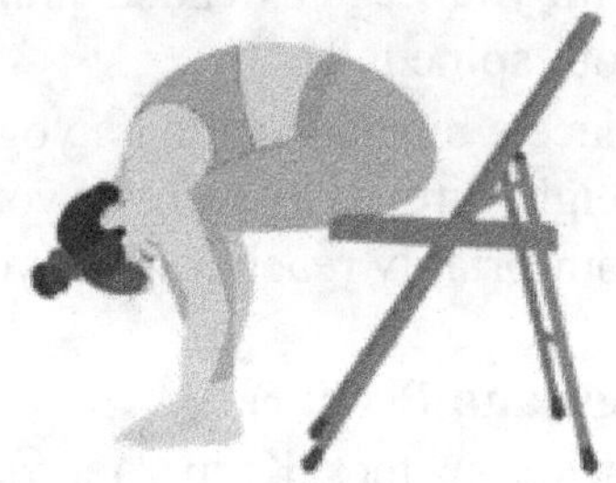

Lengthen Your Spine
- Inhale deeply to establish the length of your spine.

Hinge at Your Hips
- Exhale and tip from your hips as much as you can, keeping a straight back.
- When you reach your maximum forward fold, carefully allow your spine to round forward.

Arm Position
- Bring your arms down between your legs.
- Option 1: Push your palms firmly into the floor with your arms straight, lengthening from your pubic bone to your collarbones.
- Option 2: Press your elbows into your inner thighs to create more widening and lengthening of your inner leg muscles.

Breathe and Hold
- Stay in the pose for one to two minutes, breathing deeply and evenly.

Release the Pose
- Inhale and come up, keeping your back relaxed and using your hands on your knees to assist if your lower back feels vulnerable.
- For increased back strength, try coming up with a straight back.

Starting Position
- Sit on the floor: Begin in Dandasana (Staff Pose) with your legs extended straight in front of you and your spine tall.
- Place a block: Position a yoga block on its lowest height directly in front of your legs, where you can comfortably reach it when you fold forward.

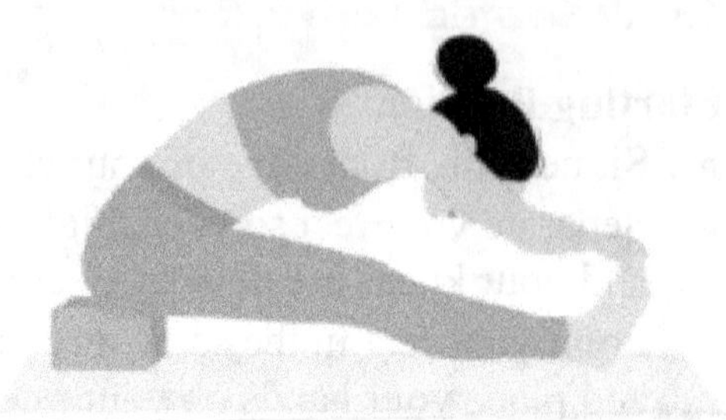

Engage and Prepare
- Flex your feet: Keep your toes pointing up toward the ceiling and your legs active.
- Inhale deeply: Lengthen through your spine, lifting your torso up and creating space between each vertebra.

Fold Forward
- Exhale: Hinge at your hips, not your waist, as you begin to fold forward. Reach your hands toward the block.
- Rest your hands on the block: Place your palms or fingertips on the block for support. Adjust the height of the block to suit your flexibility.

Deepen the Stretch
- Inhale: Lengthen your spine further, drawing your chest slightly forward.
- Exhale: Relax into the fold, allowing your head and neck to release, and deepen the stretch in your hamstrings and lower back.

Hold the Pose
- Breathe deeply: Maintain deep, steady breaths, holding the pose for 5-10 breaths.
- Stay relaxed: Keep your shoulders relaxed and your gaze soft.

Release the Pose
- Inhale: Slowly lift your torso back up, coming out of the forward fold.
- Exhale: Return to Dandasana, sitting tall with your legs extended.

The Cat-Cow sequence, often practiced in yoga, focuses on the spine and abdominal muscles. This movement involves flexing (Cat Pose) and extending (Cow Pose) the spine while synchronizing each movement with breath, creating a simple vinyasa that links breath to movement. It is highly effective for relieving back pain and tension.

Starting Position
- Get on your hands and knees. Place your wrists under your shoulders and your knees under your hips.
- Keep your spine neutral, extending from the crown of your head to your tailbone. Look down and slightly forward to keep your neck long.

Inhale for Cow Pose (Posisi Sapi - Bitilasana)
- Curl your toes under.
- Tilt your pelvis back, lifting your tailbone.
- Let this movement flow up your spine, dropping your belly and lifting your chest.
- Look up gently towards the ceiling, keeping your neck relaxed.

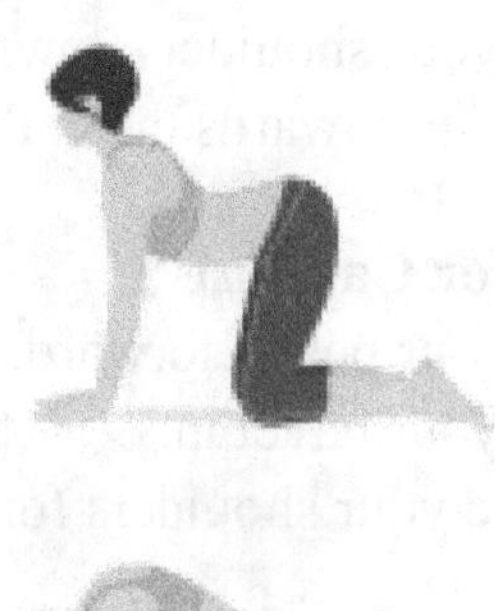

Exhale for Cat Pose (Posisi Kucing - Marjaryasana)
- Flatten the tops of your feet on the floor.
- Tuck your pelvis under, rounding your spine.
- Draw your belly towards your spine and let your head drop, looking at your navel.

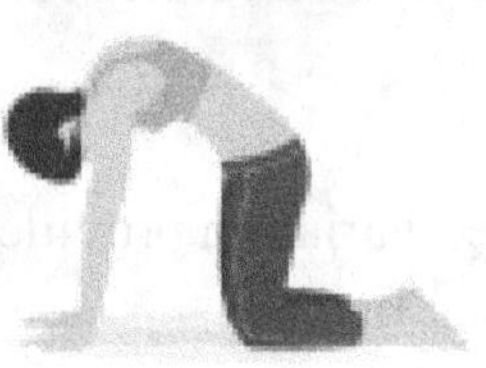

Inhale as you move into Cow Pose, arching your back and looking up.
Exhale as you move into Cat Pose, rounding your spine and tucking your head.
Continue this flow for 5 to 10 breaths, matching your movements to your breath.

Key Points
- When lifting your gaze to the ceiling, do so with control to avoid overextending your neck.
- In Cat Pose, let your head drop naturally instead of forcing it down.
- Keep your shoulders relaxed and avoid drawing them up towards your ears.
- Ensure your arms remain straight so the movement originates from your spine rather than your arms and elbows.

Variation:

If you have difficulty or limited mobility, try this seated version:

Starting Position

- Sit in a chair with your feet flat on the floor and hands on your knees.

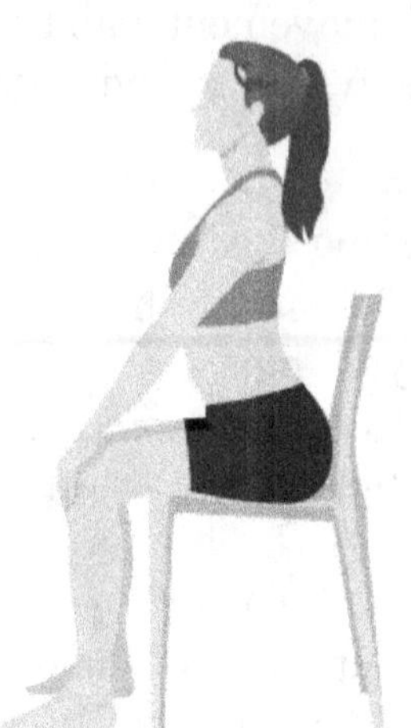

Inhale for Cow Pose

- Tilt your pelvis back, arching your lower back.
- Pull your shoulders down and back.
- Look up towards the ceiling.

Exhale for Cat Pose

- Tilt your pelvis forward, rounding your spine.
- Pull your navel in.
- Curve your shoulders forward and look towards your belly.

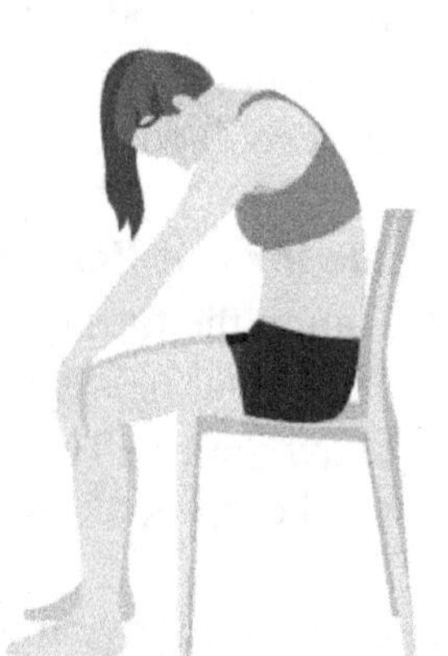

Repeat

This seated variation provides a gentle alternative while delivering similar benefits.

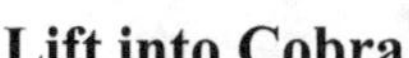

Cobra Pose, or Bhujangasana, is a rejuvenating backbend that stretches the spine, opens the chest, and strengthens the back muscles. This pose is often included in Sun Salutations and is an excellent way to counteract the effects of prolonged sitting. Practicing Cobra Pose can improve posture, relieve stress, and invigorate the body by enhancing the flow of energy. It is a fundamental pose for developing flexibility and strength in the spine, making it suitable for practitioners of all levels.

Starting Position

- Lie face down on your mat with your legs extended straight back and the tops of your feet pressing into the mat.
- Place your hands under your shoulders, palms flat on the floor, and your elbows close to your body.

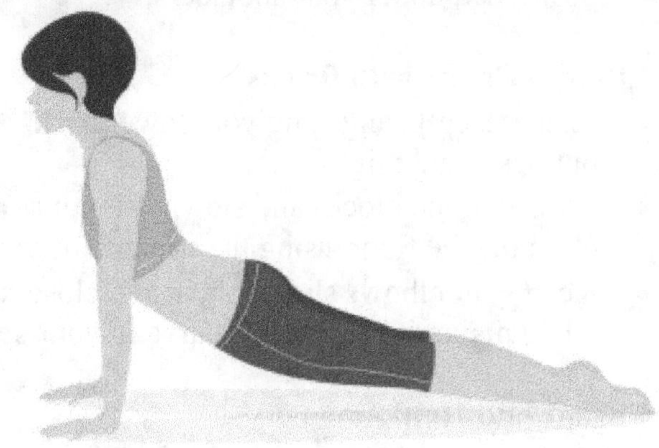

Lift into Cobra

- Inhale deeply, engaging your lower back, buttocks, and thighs.
- Press into your hands and slowly lift your chest off the floor, using the strength of your back rather than pushing with your arms.
- Keep your elbows slightly bent and close to your body, and lift only as high as comfortable while maintaining a gentle curve in your spine.

Engage and Hold

- Draw your shoulder blades back and down, opening your chest.
- Keep your gaze slightly forward or directly in front of you, avoiding any strain on your neck.
- Breathe deeply and steadily, holding the pose for 15 to 30 seconds.

Release the Pose

- Exhale and slowly lower your chest back to the floor.
- Rest your head on your hands or turn your head to one side and relax completely.

Key Points

- Use the strength of your back rather than your arms to lift your chest.
- Draw your shoulder blades back and down to create space in the chest and lungs.
- Avoid overextending your lower back by lifting only as high as comfortable.

Variations:

Starting Position

- Lie face down on your mat with your legs extended straight back and the tops of your feet pressing into the mat.
- Place two yoga blocks under your palms, positioned under your shoulders.

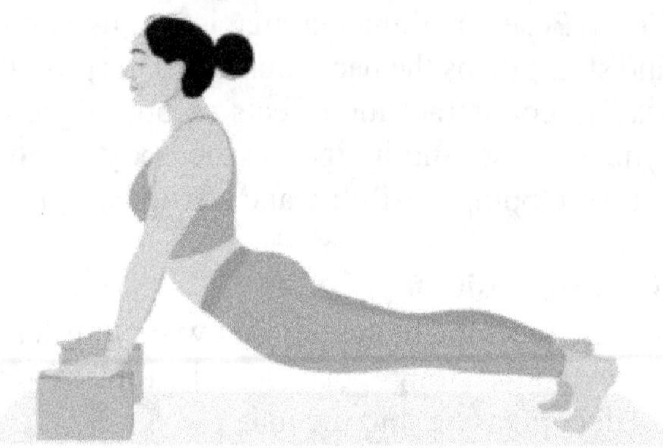

Lift into Cobra with Bricks

- Inhale deeply, engaging your lower back, buttocks, and thighs.
- Press into the blocks and slowly lift your chest off the floor, using the strength of your back and the support of the blocks.
- Keep your elbows slightly bent and close to your body, and lift only as high as comfortable while maintaining a gentle curve in your spine.

Engage and Hold

- Draw your shoulder blades back and down, opening your chest.
- Keep your gaze slightly forward or directly in front of you, avoiding any strain on your neck.
- Breathe deeply and steadily, holding the pose for 15 to 30 seconds.

Release the Pose

- Exhale and slowly lower your chest back to the floor.
- Rest your head on your hands or turn your head to one side and relax completely.

Starting Position
- Lie face down on your mat with your legs extended straight back and the tops of your feet pressing into the mat.
- Place your hands under your shoulders, palms flat on the floor, and your elbows close to your body.

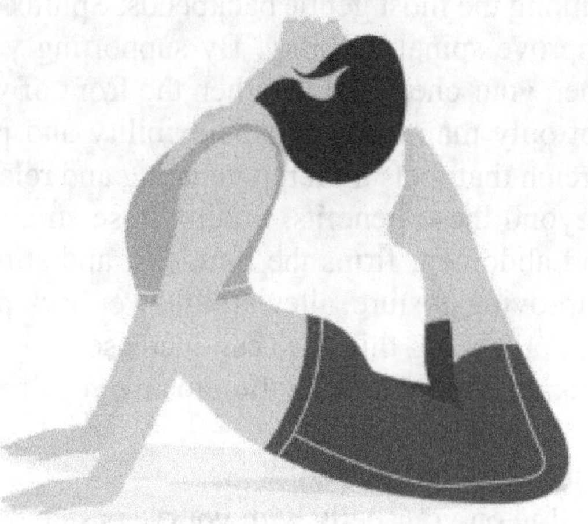

Lift into Cobra
- Inhale deeply, engaging your lower back, buttocks, and thighs.
- Press into your hands and slowly lift your chest off the floor, using the strength of your back.
- Keep your elbows slightly bent and close to your body.

Deepen into King Cobra
- Walk your hands back slightly to bring your hands closer to your waist.
- Inhale deeply, lifting your chest higher and beginning to lift your hips off the floor.
- Press the tops of your feet firmly into the mat and bend your knees, bringing your feet toward your head.

Hold the Pose
- Reach back with your head to try and meet your feet, opening your chest deeply.
- Keep your shoulder blades drawn down and back.
- Breathe deeply and steadily, holding the pose for 15 to 30 seconds.

Release the Pose
- Exhale and slowly lower your chest and legs back to the floor.
- Rest your head on your hands or turn your head to one side and relax completely.

Among the most gentle backbends, Sphinx Pose offers an excellent way to build back muscles and improve spinal mobility. By supporting yourself on your forearms and elbows, you can gently open your chest and lengthen the front of your body from the pelvic bones to the chin. This pose not only maintains spinal flexibility and promotes a healthy back but also provides a soothing stretch that feels both rejuvenating and relaxing.

Beyond these benefits, Sphinx Pose strengthens the spine, stretches the chest, lungs, shoulders, and abdomen, firms the buttocks, and stimulates abdominal organs. It is particularly useful for improving posture, alleviating lower back pain, and relieving stress. Traditional texts even suggest that practicing this pose can increase body heat, destroy disease, and awaken Kundalini's energy, making it a holistic addition to any yoga routine.

Starting Position

- Lie on your belly with your legs side by side.
- Firm your tailbone towards your pubis and lengthen it towards your heels.
- To protect your lower back, roll the outside of your thighs toward the floor and rotate your legs inward.

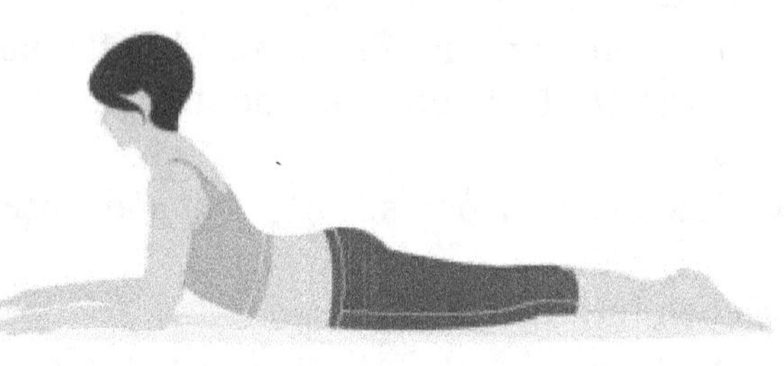

Activate Your Legs

- Reach actively through your toes towards the wall behind you.
- Continue lengthening your tail towards your heels to protect your lower back.
- Keep your buttocks firm but not clenched, and relax your tongue, eyes, and brain.

Inhale and Lift

- Set your elbows under your shoulders and forearms parallel to the floor.
- Take a deep breath in and lift your upper body and head off the ground into a mild backbend.

Engage Your Core

- Lightly draw your lower belly (just above the pubic bone) away from the floor, creating a subtle dome towards your lower back.
- This supports and distributes the curvature of your backbend evenly along your spine.

Hold the Pose

- Stay in this position for five to 10 breaths.
- Inhale deeply to broaden your back, and exhale to release any tension.

Release the Pose

- As you progressively let go of your abdomen, lower your body and lower your head to the floor, exhale.
- Gently tilt your head to one side and find a moment of stillness. As you breathe in, gently expand your back and let go of any tension as you exhale.

- Repeat the pose once or twice more if desired, allowing your body to rest between repetitions.

Key Points
- Keep your spine long and maintain a gentle curve.
- Lightly draw your lower belly away from the floor.
- Ensure elbows are directly under shoulders.

Variation:

Starting Position
- Place your feet hip-width apart and stand facing a wall.
- Brace yourself by leaning your elbows at a 90-degree angle and placing your forearms on the wall at shoulder height.

Align Your Spine
- Walk your feet back a few inches so your body forms a slight angle with the wall.
- Keep your spine long and your shoulders relaxed.

Engage Your Core
- Lightly draw your lower belly in and up to support your spine.
- Maintain a gentle engagement in your core muscles.

Inhale and Lift
- Inhale and gently press your forearms into the wall.
- Lift your chest slightly away from the wall, creating a mild backbend.

Hold the Pose
- Hold this position for five to 10 breaths.
- Focus on keeping your spine long, and your shoulders relaxed.

Release the Pose
- Return your chest to its starting position slowly as you exhale.
- Step forward to come back to an upright stance.

This variation of Sphinx Pose is particularly beneficial for those who need a gentle backbend with additional support, such as beginners, individuals with lower back pain, or anyone needing a more accessible option.

Child's Pose (Balasana)

Child's Pose (Balasana) is a foundational yoga posture that serves as the ultimate resting pose. It offers a gentle stretch for the shoulders, back, hips, thighs, neck, and ankles, providing a moment to pause, reassess, and reconnect with your breath. This pose can be particularly calming and relaxing, helping to manage stress by activating the relaxation response (parasympathetic nervous system) and deactivating the stress response (sympathetic nervous system). Regular practice of Child's Pose may help lower or regulate blood pressure, promoting overall well-being.

Starting Position

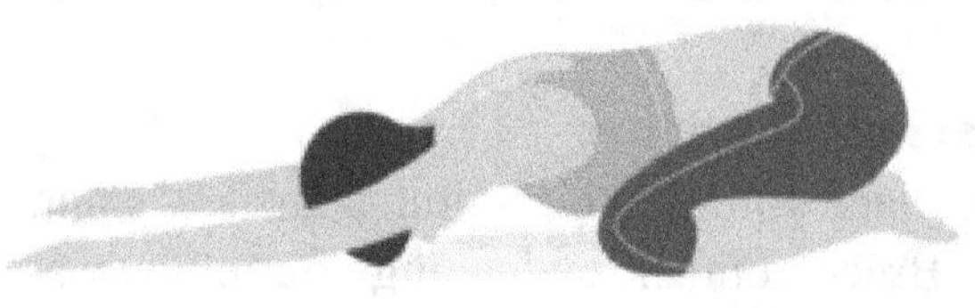

- Begin on your hands and knees on the yoga mat.
- Spread your knees wide, aligning them with the edges of your mat, and Make sure the tops of your feet are on the ground and your big toes touch.

Lower Your Body

- Exhale and sit back on your heels, then fold forward to rest your belly between your thighs.
- Root your forehead on the floor. If this is uncomfortable, use a block or stack your fists to support your forehead.

Arm Position

- Bring your shoulders and back into a straight line by extending your arms forward, palms down.
- Alternatively, extend your arms back alongside your thighs with palms facing up for a more relaxed position.

Breathing and Relaxation

- Inhale deeply, feeling the breath expand your back and ribs.
- Exhale and relax your shoulders, jaw, and eyes. Allow your body to sink into the pose.
- Stay in this position for 30 seconds to a few minutes, focusing on deep, steady breaths.

Adjust Your Position

- Broaden your sacrum and lengthen your tailbone away from your lower back.
- To make the stretch more noticeable, tuck your chin ever-so-slightly to elevate your head somewhat off the back of your neck.

Release the Pose

- To come out of the pose, inhale and slowly lengthen your torso forward.
- Exhale as you lift from your tailbone, bringing your body back to a seated position.

Repeat Child's Pose as often as needed throughout your practice. It can be particularly useful after intense sequences or challenging poses.

Key points
- Spread knees wide, big toes touching, belly between thighs.
- Ensure the forehead is comfortably supported (floor, block, or fists).
- Focus on deep, steady breaths to enhance relaxation.

Variation:

Starting Position
- Begin on your hands and knees on the yoga mat.
- Sit back on your heels as your knees are slightly apart or together, bringing your big toes together.

Lower Your Body
- Exhale and fold forward, resting your belly on your thighs and your forehead on the mat.

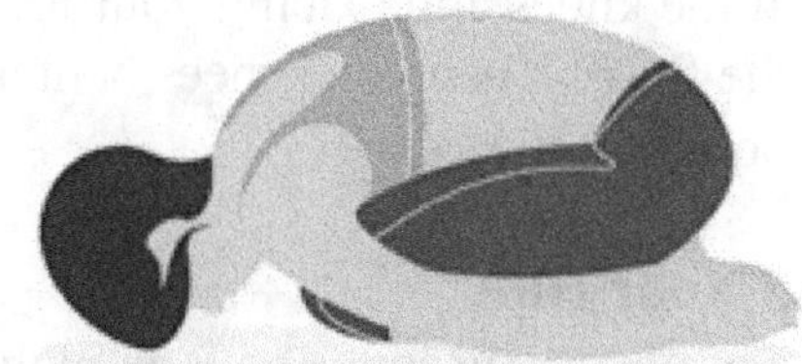

Arm Position
- Reach your arms back beside your body with the palms facing up.
- Allow your shoulders to relax and your shoulder blades to spread wide across your back.

Breathing and Relaxation
- Inhale deeply, expanding your back and ribs.
- Exhale and relax your shoulders, jaw, and eyes. Let your body sink into the pose.
- Stay in this position for 30 seconds to a few minutes, focusing on deep, steady breaths.

Release the Pose
- To come out of the pose, inhale and slowly lift your torso.
- Exhale as you bring your body back to an upright position.

This variation of Child's Pose enhances relaxation and stretches the shoulders, making it an excellent choice for relieving tension and promoting calmness.

Spinal Twist, also known as Supta Matsyendrasana, is a relaxing pose often practiced during the cool-down portion of a yoga session. This pose helps stretch the glutes, chest, and obliques, providing a deep twist that counteracts the effects of prolonged sitting. It also serves as a heart opener, improving spinal mobility and aiding digestion. Prioritizing the contact of your shoulders with the mat over your knees can deepen the Twist's effectiveness. Experimenting with this pose at different times in your practice can reveal how warmed muscles enhance stretch and relaxation.

Starting Position
- Lie down on your back.
- Get into a lying down position by bending at the knees and placing your feet flat on the floor. Keep your knees bent and pointed upwards.

Shift Your Hips
- To move your hips about an inch to the right, press into your feet to lift them off the floor a little.
- This sets your hips up to stack one on top of the other during the Twist.

Draw Your Knee In
- Let out a breath and bring your right knee up to your chest.
- Lay your left leg out flat on the floor and keep your left foot actively bent.

Inhale deeply.
- Move into the Twist
- Take a deep breath out, and then cross your right knee over your left knee to the floor on the left side of your body.
- Your right hip will now be stacked on top of your left hip.
- If it feels good, you can hook your right foot behind your left knee.

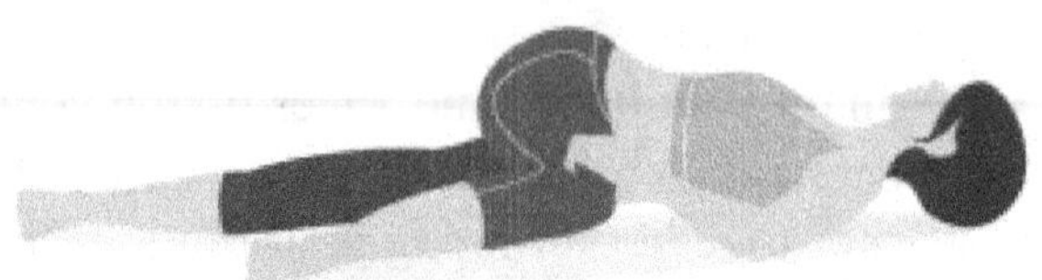

Position Your Arms
- Hold your right arm straight out to the right and open it to the right.
- Place your left hand on your right knee or spread it out in a T shape so that the palms of your hands are faced up.

Turn Your Head
- Look over your right shoulder to your right fingers as you turn your head to the right.
- Skip this step if it doesn't feel good on your neck.

Deepen the Stretch
- Let go of your left knee and your right arm toward the floor every time you exhale.
- Hold the pose for five to 10 breaths.

Release the Pose
- Roll onto your back while inhaling and bringing your right knee to your chest.
- Put your legs flat on the floor and take a few deep breaths to center your spine.

Switch Sides
- Repeat the pose on the opposite side by drawing your left knee into your chest and extending your right leg.

Key Points

- Keep shoulders on the floor as much as possibe for a stable anchor and effective stretch.
- Align hips correctly by shifting them slightly to the side before twisting.
- Turn your head gently, and only if comfortable, avoid neck strain.

Variation:

Starting Position

- Sit down on the ground and stretch your legs out straight in front of you.
- Bend your right knee and place your right foot on the outside of your left thigh.
- Stretch out your left leg, bend your left knee, and put your left foot close to your right hip.

Align Your Spine

- As you breathe in, stretch your back and sit up straight.
- Ground both sitting bones into the floor.

Move into the Twist

- Exhale and twist your torso to the right.
- Place your right hand on the floor behind you for support.
- Wrap your left arm around your right knee and hug it, or put your left elbow on the outside of your right knee for a greater twist.

Position Your Head

- Turn your head to the right, looking over your right shoulder if comfortable.
- Keep your neck relaxed and avoid straining.

Deepen the Stretch

- Inhale to lengthen your spine further.
- Exhale and deepen the twist, rotating from your belly and chest.
- Hold the pose for five to ten breaths, making sure your shoulders are relaxed and your back straight.

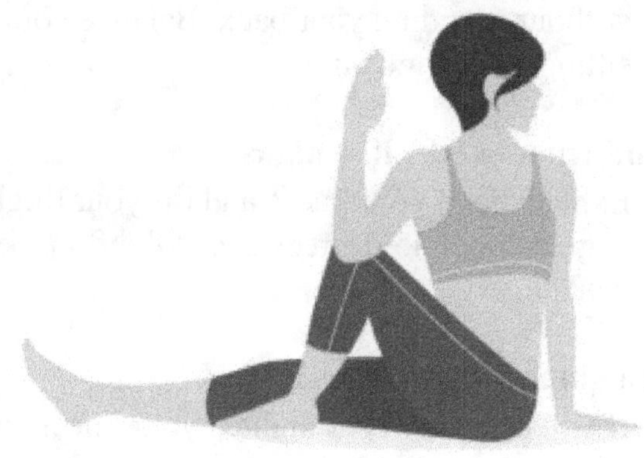

Release the Pose

- Inhale and slowly untwist your torso, returning to the starting position.
- Extend both legs straight in front of you to neutralize your spine.

Switch Sides

- Bend your left knee and put your left foot on the outside of your right thigh to make the move again on the other side.

Boat Pose (Navasana) is often associated with building strong abdominal muscles, but its benefits extend beyond just core strength. This pose also strengthens the hip flexors, adductors, and lower back muscles, which are crucial for supporting the spine. Additionally, Boat Pose offers a mental challenge, requiring focus and perseverance to maintain the posture while engaging and expanding the body. Variations of Boat Pose make it accessible to practitioners of all levels, allowing them to gradually build the necessary strength and balance to hold the pose with arms and legs fully extended.

Begin Seated
- Sit on the floor with your legs straight in front of you. Place your hands on the floor slightly behind your hips.

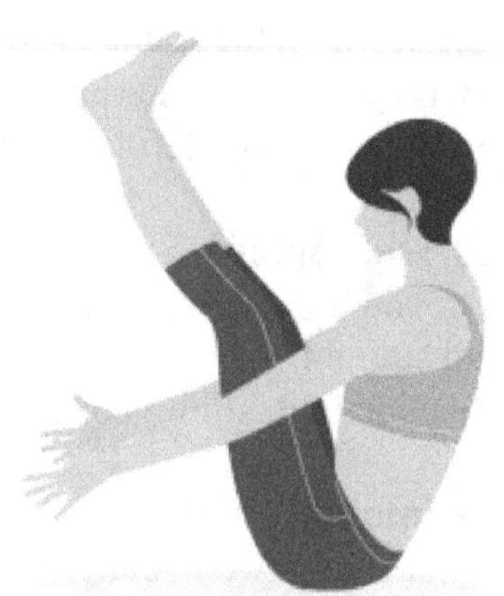

Lift Through Sternum
- Lift through the top of your sternum and lean back slightly without rounding your back. Balance your weight on your sitting bones and tailbone.

Bend Knees and Lift Thighs
- Exhale, bend your knees and lift your thighs so they are angled about 45 degrees above the floor, keeping your knees bent.

Straighten Legs (If Possible)
- If you can, slowly straighten your knees, raising the tips of your toes slightly above the level of your eyes. If not, keep your knees bent with your shins parallel to the floor.

Extend Arms Forward
- Draw your shoulders back and extend both arms forward alongside your legs, parallel to the floor, with palms facing in. Keep your lower belly flat and firm.

Hold and Breathe
- Point your toes or flex through your heels. Hold the pose for 10 to 20 seconds, gradually increasing to a minute. Maintain steady breathing throughout.

Key Points
- Focus on keeping your core engaged to support your spine and maintain balance.
- Avoid rounding your back by lifting through your sternum and keeping your spine long.
- Distribute your weight evenly on your sitting bones and tailbone to maintain balance and stability in the pose.

Variation:

Prepare to come into Boat Pose but keep your feet on
the ground.

Start Seated

- Sit on the floor with your legs straight in front of
  you. Place your hands on the floor slightly behind
  your hips.

Lift Through Sternum

- Lift through the top of your sternum and lean back
  slightly, making sure your back doesn't round.
  Balance your weight on the tripod of your sitting bones and tailbone.

Lift One Leg

- Lift one leg at a time. You can keep the lifted leg bent or straighten it.

Hold for Support

- Hold onto the back of your thighs for extra support or bring your hands behind you on the
  floor.

Transition with Breath

- Try transitioning back and forth between legs with your breath, switching legs on an
  exhalation.

Bridge Pose (Setu Bandhasana) is a versatile yoga pose that can be performed dynamically or restoratively. It serves as both a strengthener and a resting pose, offering numerous variations to suit individual needs. This pose engages all your limbs and can shift your perspective on yoga, emphasizing ease and breath over struggle. The benefits of Bridge Pose include gentle stretching of the chest, shoulders, and abdomen while strengthening the back, glutes, thighs, and ankles. It also improves posture, counteracts the effects of prolonged sitting, and may help relieve lower back pain and kyphosis. Additionally, Bridge Pose shares many benefits with conventional inversions, as it brings your head below your heart.

Starting Position

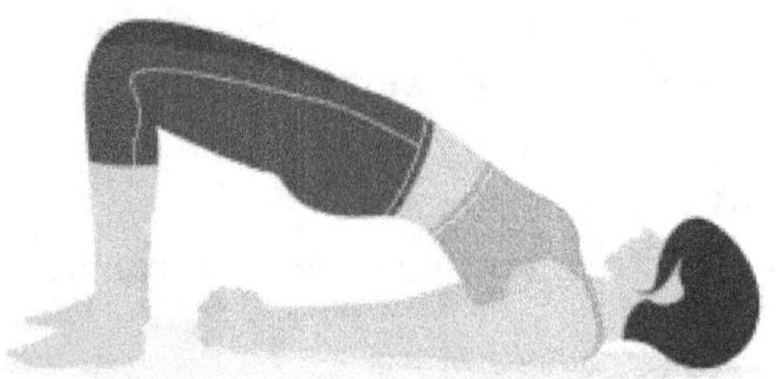

- Lie on your back with your knees bent and your feet on the mat, hip-distance apart. Inch your feet as close to your glutes as possible.
- Bring your arms alongside your body, palms down.

Lift Hips

- As you inhale, press down firmly through your feet and lift your hips, initiating the movement from the pubic bone.

Engage Arms

- Press your upper arms down. You can clasp your hands behind your back and press your pinkie fingers into the mat. Broaden your collarbones and roll your shoulders beneath you.

Align Body

- Press down firmly through your heels, draw your thighs toward one another to keep them hip-distance apart, and reach the backs of your thighs toward your knees to lengthen your spine.

Hold and Breathe

- Stay in this pose for 5 to 15 breaths.

Release the Pose

- Exhale as you release your hands and slowly lower yourself to the mat.

Key Points

- Press the inner feet down and engage the inner thighs to keep the knees from splaying out.

- Lengthen the tailbone and keep the neck neutral by sliding the shoulder blades down the back.
- Coordinate the lift of the hips with your inhalation and lower the spine with your exhalation.

Variation:

Supported Bridge Pose (Setu Bandhasana with Support)

Starting Position
- Lie on your back: Begin by lying flat on your back with your knees bent and feet flat on the floor, hip-width apart. Your arms should be resting alongside your body, palms facing down.
- Place a block: Position a yoga block within reach, near your hips.

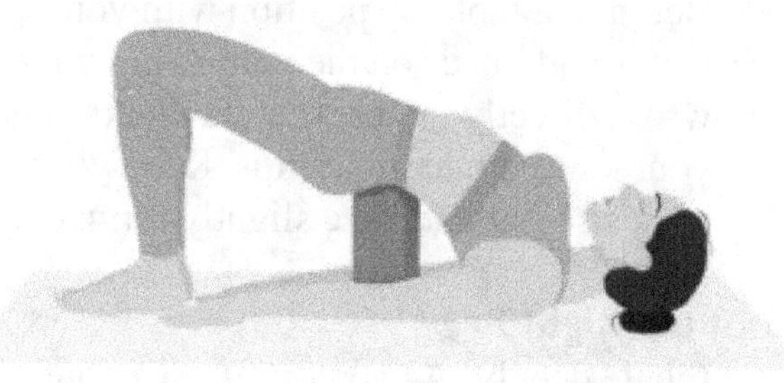

Engage and Prepare
- Adjust your feet: Make sure your feet are parallel and close enough to your hips that your fingertips can just touch your heels.
- Inhale deeply: Press your feet firmly into the floor and lift your hips slightly, creating a gentle arch in your lower back.

Lift and Support
- Exhale: Press through your feet and lift your hips off the ground, creating a bridge shape with your body.
- Place the block: Slide the yoga block under your sacrum (the flat part of your lower back) for support. Adjust the height of the block (low, medium, or high) to suit your comfort level.

Find Stability
- Rest your hips: Allow your hips to rest fully on the block, ensuring it feels stable and supportive.
- Position your arms: You can keep your arms alongside your body or interlace your fingers underneath your back for a deeper stretch, pressing your arms into the floor.

Hold the Pose
- Breathe deeply: Take deep, steady breaths, allowing your chest to expand and your abdomen to rise and fall with each inhale and exhale.
- Stay relaxed: Keep your neck relaxed and your gaze directed toward the ceiling. Hold the pose for 5-10 breaths, or longer if comfortable.

Release the Pose
- Inhale: Press your feet onto the floor, lift your hips slightly, and remove the block.
- Exhale: Slowly lower your hips back down to the floor, one vertebra at a time.
- Rest: Bring your knees together and your feet wide apart, allowing your back to relax for a few breaths.

Tiger Pose (Vyaghrasana) is a dynamic yoga pose that mimics the graceful and powerful movements of a tiger. This pose is excellent for building strength and flexibility in the spine, hips, and shoulders. It also helps to improve balance and coordination while providing a gentle stretch for the back and chest. Practicing Tiger Pose can invigorate your body, enhance your focus, and release tension in the lower back and hips.

Starting Position
- Begin in a tabletop position with your hands and knees on the mat. Align your wrists directly under your shoulders and your knees under your hips. Keep your back straight and gaze slightly forward.

Lift the Right Leg
- Inhale deeply. As you exhale, lift your right leg off the mat and extend it straight back. Keep your foot flexed and your leg parallel to the floor. Engage your core to maintain balance.

Bend the Right Knee
- Inhale, bend your right knee and bring your heel towards your buttocks. Keep your thigh parallel to the floor and maintain the alignment of your hips.

Lift the Left Arm
- As you exhale, lift your left arm off the mat and extend it straight forward. Your arm should be parallel to the floor, and your fingers should point forward. Keep your gaze slightly forward to help with balance.

Hold the Pose
- Hold this position for a few breaths, maintaining a steady and balanced posture. Feel the stretch along your spine and the engagement of your core, shoulders, and hips.

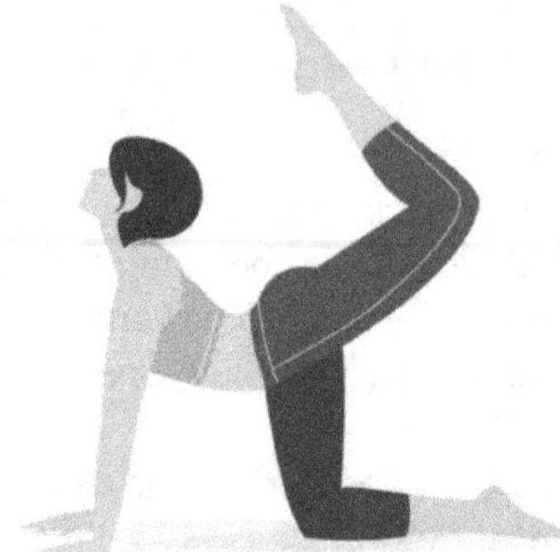

Return to the Tabletop Position
- Inhale, lower your left arm and right leg back to the mat, returning to the tabletop position. Take a moment to stabilize and prepare for the other side.

Repeat on the Other Side
- Repeat the steps by lifting your left leg and right arm, maintaining balance and focus. Hold the pose for an equal amount of time on each side.

Complete the Pose
- After completing both sides, return to the tabletop position and take a few deep breaths to relax your muscles and release any tension.

Key Points
- Engage Core: Keep core muscles active for balance and lower back protection.
- Maintain Alignment: Wrists under shoulders, knees under hips, arm and leg parallel to the floor.
- Breathe Steadily: Inhale deeply while lifting, exhale fully while holding.

Camel Pose, or Ustrasana, is a backbend that opens the chest, stretches the entire front of the body, and strengthens the back muscles. This pose is excellent for improving flexibility in the spine and is often used as a heart-opening posture to counteract the effects of forward slumping from prolonged sitting. Performing Camel Pose requires both strength and flexibility, making it a potent pose for deepening your practice.

Starting Position
- Begin by kneeling on your mat with your knees hip-width apart and your thighs perpendicular to the floor. Place your hands on your lower back with your fingers pointing down.

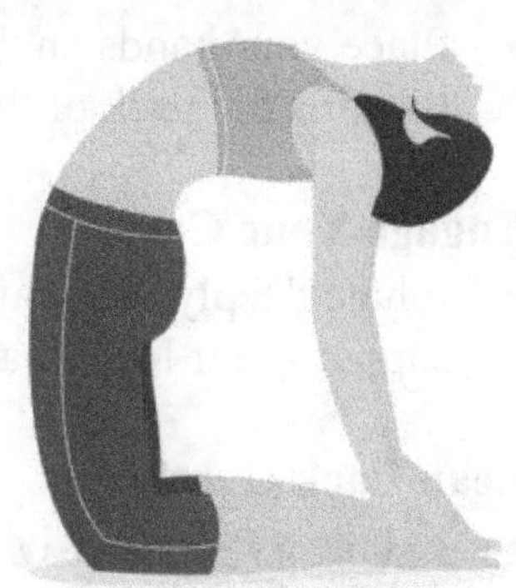

Engage Your Core
- Inhale deeply, lifting your chest. Engage your core muscles to support your lower back. Tuck your chin slightly toward your chest to lengthen the back of your neck.

Lift and Open the Chest
- Exhale as you slowly start to lean back, pressing your hips forward. Keep your hands on your lower back for support.

Reach for Your Heels
- Continue to press your hips forward as you reach your hands back to grasp your heels, one at a time. If this is too intense, keep your hands on your lower back.

Deepen the Backbend
- Once you are holding your heels, press your hips forward and lift your chest higher. Drop your head back gently if it feels comfortable, keeping your neck relaxed.

Hold the Pose
- Hold this position for 5-10 breaths, breathing deeply and evenly. Focus on lifting through your chest and keeping your core engaged to support your back.

Release the Pose
- To come out of the pose, bring your hands back to your lower back for support. Inhale as you slowly rise back up to a kneeling position, leading with your chest.

Key Points
- Keep your abdominal muscles engaged to support and protect your lower back throughout the pose.
- Focus on lifting and expanding your chest to achieve a deep, heart-opening stretch.
- Continuously press your hips forward to deepen the backbend and maintain proper alignment.

Variations:

Starting Position
- Kneel in front of a chair with the seat facing you. Your knees should be hip-width apart, and your thighs perpendicular to the floor.

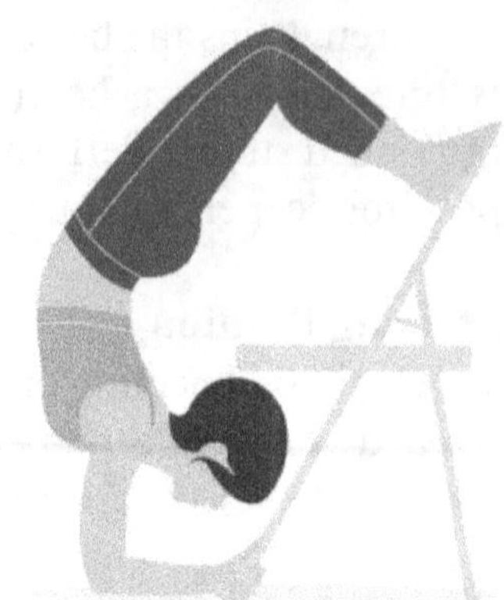

Place Hands on the Chair
- Place your hands on the chair seat with your fingers pointing towards the back of the chair.

Engage Your Core
- Inhale deeply, lift your chest and engage your core muscles to support your lower back.

Lean Back Gently
- Exhale as you slowly start to lean back, pressing your hips forward while keeping your hands on the chair for support.

Deepen the Backbend
- Walk your hands back along the chair seat, or hold the sides or back of the chair as you deepen the backbend. Continue to press your hips forward and lift through your chest.

Hold the Pose
- Hold this position for 5-10 breaths, breathing deeply and evenly. Focus on the support of the chair to maintain your alignment.

Release the Pose
- To come out of the pose, walk your hands forward on the chair to return to an upright kneeling position. Inhale as you slowly rise back up, leading with your chest.

Starting Position
- Kneel in front of a chair with the seat facing away from you. Your knees should be hip-width apart, and your thighs perpendicular to the floor.

Place Hands on Chair Legs
- Place your hands on the back legs of the chair for support.

Engage Your Core
- Inhale deeply, lift your chest and engage your core muscles to support your lower back.

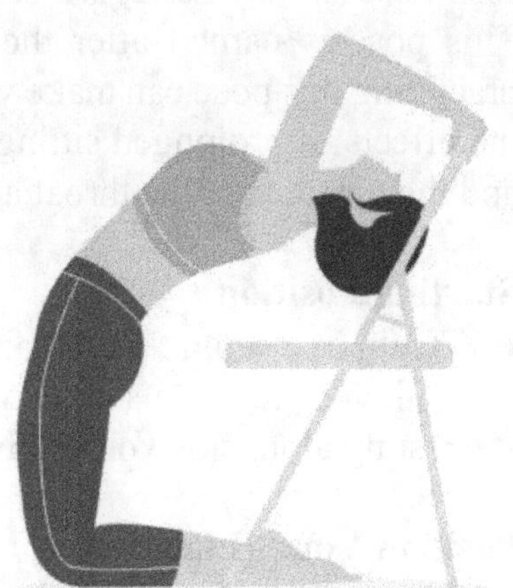

Lean Back and Rest Head
- Exhale as you slowly start to lean back, pressing your hips forward. Continue leaning until your head gently rests on the chair seat.

Hold the Pose
- Hold this position for 5-10 breaths, breathing deeply and evenly. Focus on the support of the chair to maintain your alignment.

Release the Pose
- To come out of the pose, use your hands to push against the chair legs, lifting your head off the chair seat. Inhale as you slowly rise back up to an upright kneeling position.

Fish Pose (Matsyasana) is a back-bending yoga posture that opens the chest, throat, and abdomen. This pose is named after the Sanskrit word "Matsya," which means fish. It is believed that practicing this pose can make you float like a fish in water. Fish Pose is excellent for counteracting the effects of prolonged sitting and poor posture. It stretches the hip flexors, intercostal muscles, and the muscles of the throat and neck while strengthening the upper back muscles.

Starting Position
- Begin in a supine position: Lie on your back with your legs extended and your arms resting alongside your body.

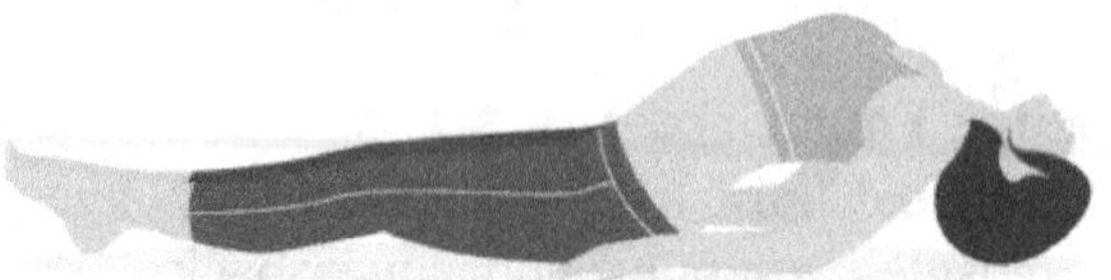

Position Your Hands
- Place your hands under your hips: Slide your hands, palms down, under your buttocks to support your lower back. Ensure your elbows are close to your torso.

Prepare for the Pose
- Lift your chest: Press your forearms and elbows firmly into the floor. As you inhale, lift your chest toward the ceiling, creating an arch in your upper back.
- Tilt your head back: Gently tilt your head back, allowing the crown of your head to rest lightly on the floor. Avoid putting too much weight on your head to prevent neck strain.

Engage Your Legs
- Activate your legs: Keep your legs strong and active, pressing your thighs and heels into the floor.

Hold the Pose
- Breathe deeply: Hold the pose for 5-10 deep breaths, feeling the stretch in your chest, throat, and abdomen.

Release the Pose
- Lower your chest: To release, press firmly into your forearms and elbows again, lift your head slightly, and lower your chest and head back to the floor.
- Relax: Remove your hands from under your buttocks and relax your arms alongside your body.

Key Points
- Focus on lifting and opening your chest to deepen the backbend and stretch the intercostal muscles.
- Ensure your neck is relaxed and there is minimal weight on the crown of your head to avoid strain.
- Keep your legs active and pressing into the floor to support the lower back and maintain stability.

Variations:

Starting Position
- Place a chair on your mat: Position a sturdy chair on your yoga mat with the backrest facing away from you.

Sit on the Chair
- Sit on the edge: Sit on the edge of the chair, facing away from the backrest. Ensure your feet are flat on the floor and your knees are bent at a 90-degree angle.

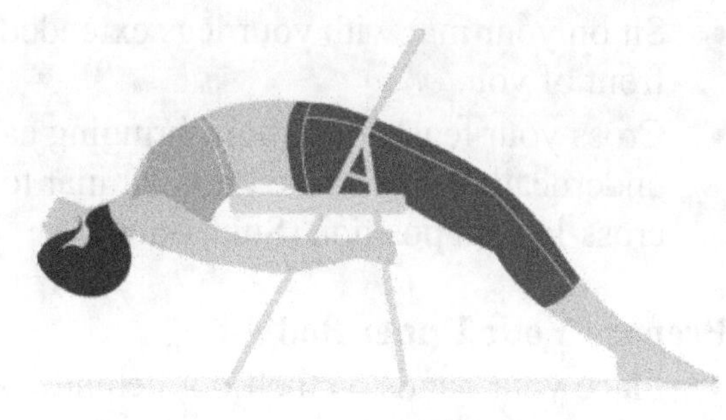

Position Your Hands
- Hold the chair: Place your hands on the sides of the chair seat for support.

Lean Back
- Lean back slowly: Gently lean back, allowing your upper back to rest on the backrest of the chair. Your head and neck should extend slightly over the top of the backrest.

Open Your Chest
- Lift your chest: Lift and open your chest, creating an arch in your upper back. Let your shoulders relax and drop toward the floor.

Engage Your Legs
- Activate your legs: Keep your legs strong and active with your feet firmly planted on the floor.

Hold the Pose
- Breathe deeply: Hold the pose for 5-10 deep breaths, focusing on the stretch in your chest, throat, and abdomen.

Release the Pose
- Return to upright: To release, use your hands to gently push yourself back to an upright seated position on the chair.
- Relax: Sit comfortably and take a few deep breaths to relax and center yourself.

Starting Position
- Sit on your mat with your legs extended straight in front of you.
- Cross your legs at the shins, bringing each foot underneath the opposite knee, similar to a seated cross-legged position (Sukhasana).

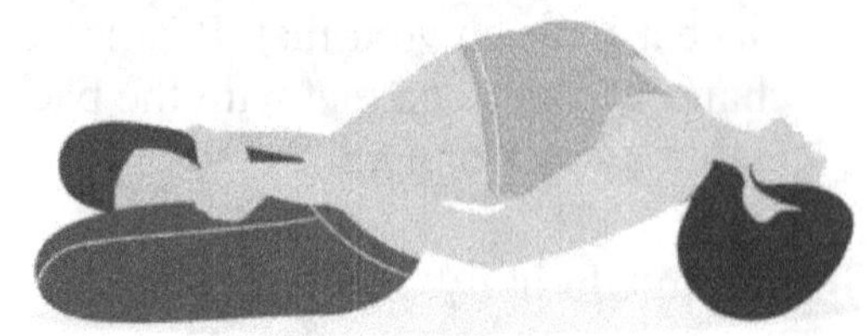

Prepare Your Upper Body
- Place your hands on the floor behind you with your fingers pointing toward your feet.
- Press your hands into the mat, and as you inhale, lift your chest toward the ceiling, allowing your back to arch.

Lower Your Head
- Slowly lower your head back towards the mat.
- Gently rest the crown of your head on the mat, keeping a slight arch in your upper back.

Position Your Arms
- Release your hands from the mat and extend your arms alongside your body with palms facing upward.
- Alternatively, you can place your hands on your thighs.

Adjust Your Legs
- Ensure that your legs remain comfortably crossed.
- If you feel any strain in your hips or knees, adjust the cross of your legs or place a folded blanket under your hips for added support.

Breathe and Hold
- Breathe deeply and evenly, focusing on opening your chest and maintaining the gentle arch on your back.
- Hold the pose for 5-10 breaths, allowing your body to relax into the stretch.

Release the Pose
- To come out of the pose, gently press your hands into the mat to lift your head and upper body back to an upright seated position.
- Uncross your legs and extend them straight in front of you.

Starting Position
- Begin by sitting on your mat with your legs extended straight in front of you.

Prepare Your Upper Body
- Place your hands on the floor behind you with your fingers pointing towards your feet.
- Press your hands into the mat, and as you inhale, lift your chest toward the ceiling, allowing your back to arch slightly.

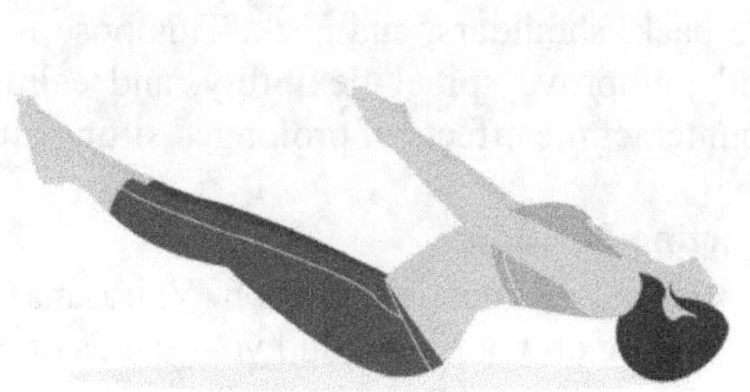

Lift Your Legs
- Lean back slightly to find balance, then lift both legs off the ground to about a 45-degree angle.
- Keep your legs together and your feet pointed.

Position Your Arms
- Extend your arms forward, parallel to the ground, with your palms facing down.
- Engage your core to help maintain balance in this position.

Arch Your Back
- Continue to lift your chest and arch your back, aiming to rest on the crown of your head.
- Ensure that your neck is long and not compressed.

Maintain the Pose
- Focus on lifting your chest and legs while keeping your core engaged.
- Breathe deeply and evenly, holding the pose for 5-10 breaths.

Release the Pose
- To come out of the pose, slowly lower your legs back to the mat and bring your upper body to an upright seated position.
- Place your hands on the mat behind you to support yourself as you sit up.

Introduction: Rabbit Pose (Sasangasana) is a gentle forward-bending posture that deeply stretches the back, shoulders, and neck. This pose is known for its ability to relieve tension in the upper body, improve spinal flexibility, and calm the mind. It's often included in yoga practices to counteract the effects of prolonged sitting and to provide a soothing stretch for the entire spine.

Starting Position
- Begin in a kneeling position (Vajrasana) with your hips resting on your heels and your hands on your thighs.

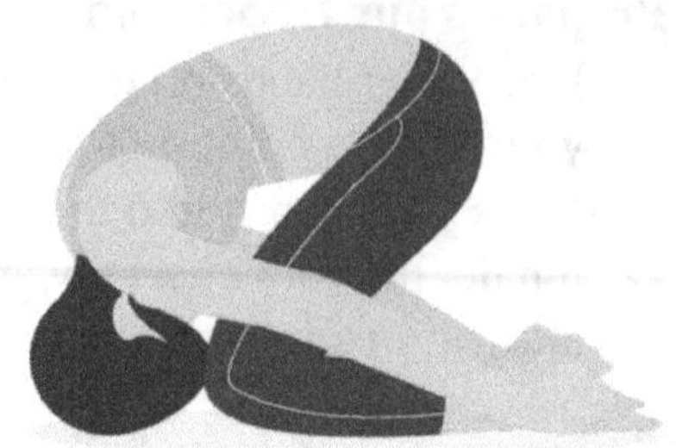

Preparation
- Inhale deeply, lengthening your spine as you prepare to move into the pose.

Grip Your Heels
- Exhale and reach back to grasp your heels with your hands, keeping your thumbs on the outside and fingers on the inside.

Tuck Your Chin
- Tuck your chin to your chest, bringing your forehead toward your knees.

Lift Your Hips
- On an inhale, lift your hips toward the ceiling while maintaining your grip on your heels. Roll onto the crown of your head, bringing your forehead as close to your knees as possible.

Deepen the Pose
- Pull on your heels gently to lift your hips higher and deepen the stretch along your spine. Keep your neck relaxed and your shoulders away from your ears.

Hold the Pose
- Stay in Rabbit Pose for 5-10 breaths, focusing on deep, steady breathing. Feel the stretch in your back and the opening of your shoulders.

Release the Pose
- To come out of the pose, release your grip on your heels and lower your hips back to your heels. Lift your head last, returning to the starting position.

Rest
- Rest in Child's Pose (Balasana) for a few breaths to relax and observe the effects of the pose.

Key Points
- Use your core muscles to support the lift of your hips and to maintain balance the pose.
- Hold your heels gently without straining your wrists or shoulders, allowing for a smooth and controlled movement.
- Focus on deep, even breaths to help deepen the stretch and to keep your body relaxed.

Locust Pose (Salabhasana)

Locust Pose, or Salabhasana, is a backbend that strengthens the muscles of the spine, buttocks, and backs of the arms and legs. This pose is excellent for improving posture, increasing flexibility in the spine, and building core strength. It provides a gentle yet effective way to counteract the effects of prolonged sitting and slouching, making it an essential addition to any yoga practice.

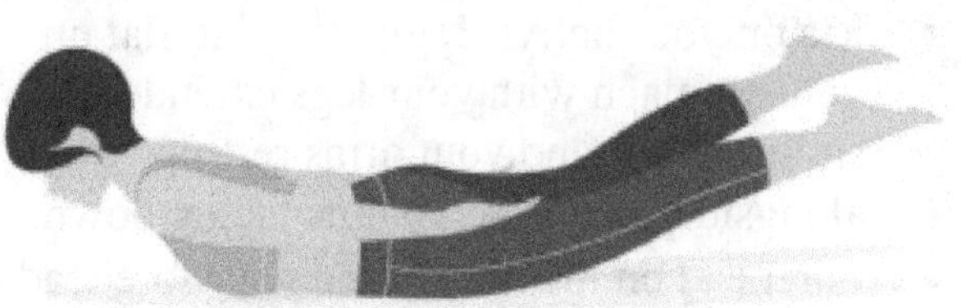

Starting Position
- **Lie on your belly:** Begin by lying flat on your stomach with your legs extended straight back and your arms resting alongside your body, palms facing down.
- **Forehead on the mat:** Place your forehead on the mat, keeping your neck in a neutral position.

Engage and Lift
- **Inhale deeply:** Engage your core and lengthen your spine, reaching through your toes and the crown of your head.
- **Lift your chest:** On your next inhale, lift your chest, arms, and legs off the mat simultaneously. Keep your arms parallel to the floor and your palms facing each other or down.
- **Engage your legs:** Press strongly through your legs, lifting them as high as possible without bending the knees. Squeeze your inner thighs together and activate your glute muscles.
- **Lengthen your spine:** Continue to lift your chest and head, extending through your spine to create a long, even arch. Keep your gaze slightly forward, maintaining a neutral neck position.

Hold the Pose
- **Breathe steadily:** Take deep, steady breaths, holding the pose for 5-10 breaths. Focus on maintaining the lift and engagement in your muscles without straining.
- **Stay strong:** Keep your arms active and parallel to the floor, reaching back through your fingertips.
- **Lengthen through your legs:** Extend through your toes and maintain the lift in your legs, keeping them straight and strong.

Release the Pose
- **Exhale and lower:** On an exhale, gently lower your chest, arms, and legs back down to the mat.
- **Rest:** Turn your head to one side and rest for a few breaths before repeating the pose or moving on to another asana.

Key Points
- Keep your abdominal muscles engaged to support your lower back and maintain the lift.

- Focus on creating length from your toes to the crown of your head, avoiding compression in the lower back.
- Breathe deeply and evenly, ensuring that you are not holding your breath while holding the pose.

Variation:

Extended Locust Pose

Starting Position
- Lie on your belly: Begin by lying flat on your stomach with your legs extended straight back and your arms resting alongside your body, palms facing down.
- Forehead on the mat: Place your forehead on the mat, keeping your neck in a neutral position.

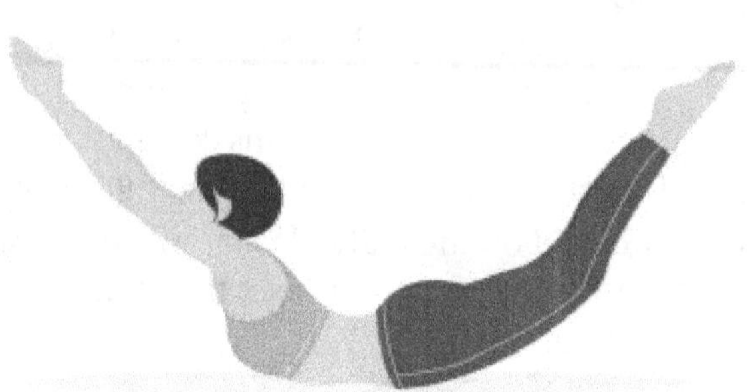

Engage and Lift
- Inhale deeply: Engage your core and lengthen your spine, reaching through your toes and the crown of your head.
- Extend your arms: Stretch your arms forward in front of you, with your palms facing each other.
- Lift your chest and legs: On your next inhale, lift your chest, arms, and legs off the mat simultaneously. Keep your arms extended forward and parallel to the floor.
- Engage your legs: Press strongly through your legs, lifting them as high as possible without bending the knees. Squeeze your inner thighs together and activate your glute muscles.
- Lengthen your spine: Continue to lift your chest and head, extending through your spine to create a long, even arch. Keep your gaze slightly forward, maintaining a neutral neck position.

Hold the Pose
- Breathe steadily: Take deep, steady breaths, holding the pose for 5-10 breaths. Focus on maintaining the lift and engagement in your muscles without straining.
- Stay strong: Keep your arms active and extended, reaching forward through your fingertips.
- Lengthen through your legs: Extend through your toes and maintain the lift in your legs, keeping them straight and strong.

Release the Pose
- Exhale and lower: On an exhale, gently lower your chest, arms, and legs back down to the mat.
- Rest: Turn your head to one side and rest for a few breaths before repeating the pose or moving on to another asana.

This variation, Extended Locust Pose, intensifies the stretch and engagement of the muscles, providing a deeper backbend and greater strengthening of the core and lower back.

One of the most well-known and fundamental yoga positions is Downward Facing Dog, also known as Adho Mukha Svanasana. It often serves as a starting point for beginners and is frequently practiced in Vinyasa yoga classes. This pose acts as both a transitional pose and a resting position, making it a cornerstone in sequences like Sun Salutation. While strengthening the external oblique abdominal muscles and stretching the hamstrings and calves, Downward Dog also strengthens the arms and legs. Additionally, as a mild inversion, it helps reverse the usual forces on the spine, promoting blood flow to the brain and potentially relieving chronic back pain when practiced regularly.

Starting Position
- Come to your hands and knees on the yoga mat.
- Assume a standing position with your hands beneath your shoulders and knees beneath your hips.

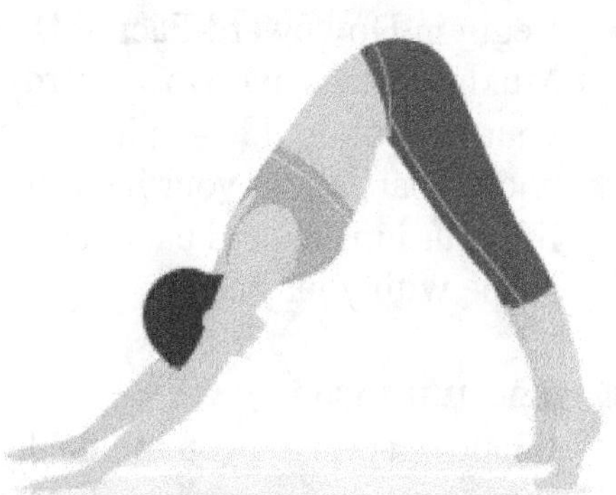

Lift Your Hips
- Curl your toes under.
- Exhale and push back through your hands to lift your hips and straighten your legs.

Hand and Arm Position
- Spread your fingers wide.
- Ground down from your forearms into your fingertips.
- Outwardly rotate your upper arms to broaden your collarbones.

Engage Your Body
- Relax your shoulders and bring them in toward your hips while you let your head droop.
- To distribute your body's weight more evenly, contract your quadriceps.

Adjust Your Legs and Feet
- Rotate your thighs inward, keep your tailbone high, and sink your heels towards the floor.
- By stepping forward into a plank position, you can check that the space between your hands and feet is correct. Both positions should maintain the same distance.

Breathe and Hold
- Inhale deeply, expanding your chest.
- Exhale, lengthening your spine and sinking your heels closer to the floor.
- Hold the pose for 5 to 10 breaths, maintaining engagement and alignment.

Release the Pose
- Exhale and bend your knees.
- Come back to your hands and knees to rest.

Key Points

- Your wrists should be under your shoulders and your knees under your hips to form a straight line.
- Contract quadriceps and core to support the body and reduce arm strain.
- Take deep, steady breaths to expand your chest and stretch your spine.

Variations:

Downward Dog Hand to Ankle

Starting Position

- Begin in Downward-Facing Dog: Start in Adho Mukha Svanasana (Downward-Facing Dog) with your hands shoulder-width apart and your feet hip-width apart. Press your heels toward the floor and lift your hips up and back, creating an inverted V-shape with your body.

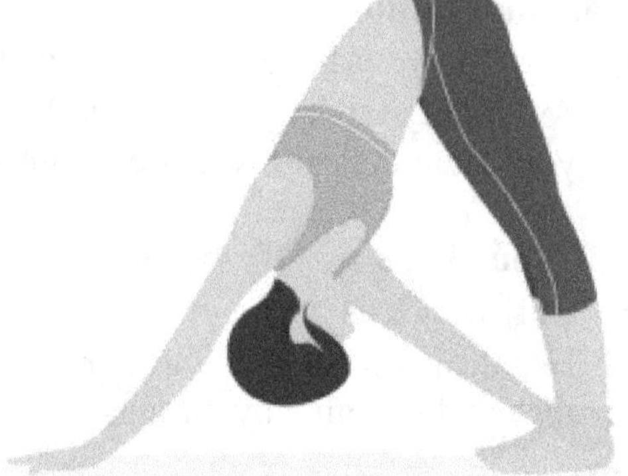

Engage and Reach

- Inhale deeply: As you inhale, lengthen through your spine, reaching your hips higher and pressing firmly into your hands and feet.
- Lift one hand: On an exhale, lift your right hand off the mat and reach it back towards your left ankle or shin. If you can reach it, lightly hold your ankle or shin.
- Twist your torso: Gently twist your torso to the left, looking underneath your left armpit. Keep your hips lifted and your legs strong.

Hold the Pose

- Breathe steadily: Take deep, steady breaths, holding the pose for 3-5 breaths. Focus on maintaining the twist and the lift in your hips without straining.
- Stay strong: Keep your supporting arm and leg active and engaged.
- Deepen the stretch: With each exhale, try to deepen the twist slightly without forcing it.

Release the Pose

- Exhale and release: On an exhale, gently release your ankle or shin and bring your right hand back to the mat, returning to Downward-Facing Dog.
- Rest: Take a few breaths in Downward-Facing Dog before repeating on the other side.

Begin in Downward Facing Dog
- Start in Downward Facing Dog with your hands shoulder-width apart and your feet hip-width apart.
- Press your hands firmly into the mat, and lift your hips towards the ceiling.

Lift One Leg
- Inhale deeply and lift your right leg towards the ceiling.
- Keep your hips squared and your lifted leg straight and strong.
- Flex your right foot and point your toes down towards the floor.

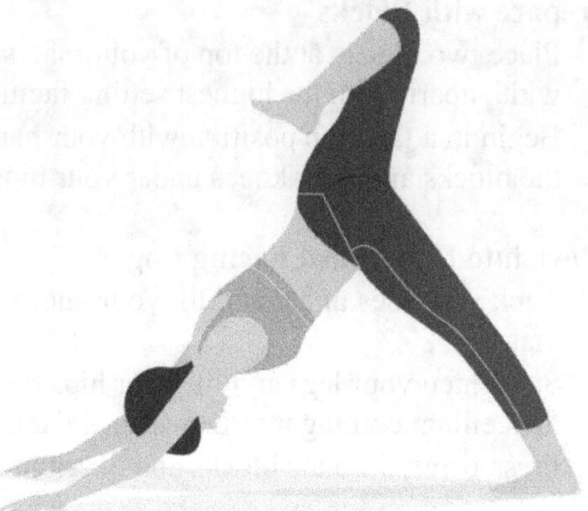

Hold the Pose
- Maintain an even weight distribution between both hands and your standing foot.
- Keep your gaze between your hands or towards your navel.
- Hold the pose for 5-10 breaths, keeping your breath steady and deep.

Return to Downward Facing Dog
- Exhale and lower your right leg back to the mat.
- Return to Downward Facing Dog and take a few breaths before repeating on the other side.

Prepare with Blocks
- Place two blocks at the top of your mat, shoulder-width apart, with the highest setting facing up.
- Begin in a tabletop position with your hands on the blocks and your knees under your hips.

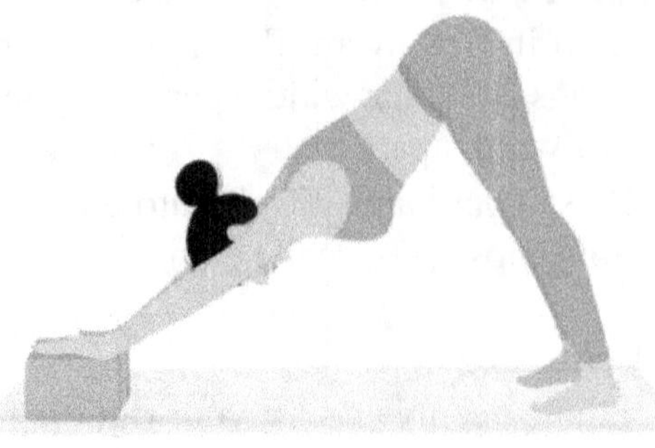

Move into Downward Facing Dog
- Tuck your toes under and lift your knees off the mat.
- Straighten your legs and lift your hips towards the ceiling, coming into Downward Facing Dog with your hands on the blocks.
- Press firmly into the blocks and distribute your weight evenly.

Adjust and Hold the Pose
- Ensure your hands are shoulder-width apart on the blocks and your feet are hip-width apart on the mat.
- Keep your spine long and your head relaxed between your arms.
- Hold the pose for 5-10 breaths, maintaining a steady and deep breathing rhythm.

Return to Starting Position
- To release the pose, gently lower your knees back to the mat.
- Sit back on your heels in Child's Pose for a few breaths to relax.

Cow Face Pose, known as Gomukhasana in Sanskrit, is a powerful yoga posture that helps rebalance the upper back and cervical region. This pose stretches the chest, shoulders, triceps, and thighs, and opens the armpits and large dorsal muscles. It also alleviates accumulated stress in the shoulders and neck, promoting a sense of relaxation and openness. The name "Gomukhasana" comes from the Sanskrit words "go" (cow) and "mukha" (face), as the pose's shape resembles a cow's face with the folded legs representing the mouth and the arms and ears. Practicing this pose on a daily basis helps improve posture, mitigate the consequences of prolonged sitting, and increase total body symmetry.

Starting Position
- Begin in Dandasana (Staff Pose) with your legs extended straight in front of you.

Position Your Legs
- Bend your knees and bring your feet to the floor.
- Slide your left foot under your right leg, placing it beside your right hip.
- Cross your right leg over your left, stacking your right knee on top of your left knee, and position your right foot beside your left hip.
- If you find it difficult to keep your back straight, sit on a yoga block or cushion.

Adjust Your Hips
- Shift your weight slightly to find balance and ensure both sitting bones are grounded.

Arm Position
- Inhale and extend your right arm out to the side, palm facing down.
- Rotate your arm inward and bend your elbow, bringing your hand to your lower back.
- Exhale and stretch your left arm up towards the ceiling, palm facing forward.
- Bend your left elbow and reach down to clasp your right hand behind your back. Use a strap if your hands do not meet.

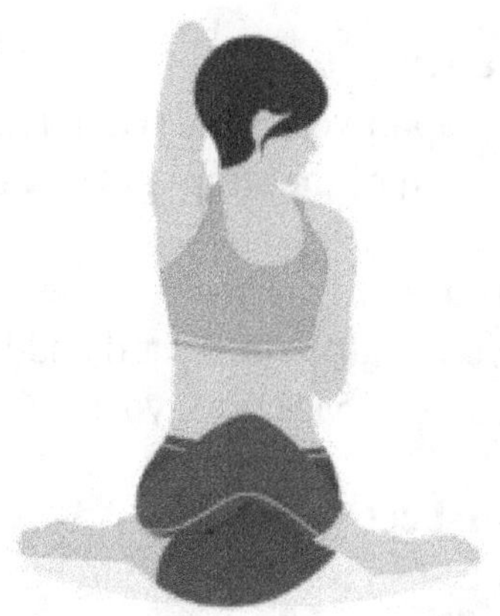

Align Your Spine
- Keep your spine straight, neck long, and chest open.
- Ensure your shoulders are aligned and pulled down away from your ears.

Breathe and Hold
- Inhale deeply to lengthen your spine.
- Exhale and deepen the stretch by gradually bringing your hands closer together.
- While holding the position, breathe deeply and evenly for 40 to 60 seconds.

Release the Pose
- Inhale and release your arms, bringing them back to your sides.
- Exhale and uncross your legs, extending them back into Dandasana.

Repeat the pose on the opposite side, with the left knee on top and the right elbow pointing upwards.

Key Points

- Ensure both sitting bones are evenly grounded.
- Use a strap if needed to connect your hands behind your back.
- Keep the spine straight and chest open.

Variation:

Cow Face Pose Variant Using a Strap (Gomukhasana)

Prepare the Strap

- Hold a strap in your right hand, reaching up with your right arm.
- Drop the end of the strap down your back.

Position Your Arms

- Rotate your right arm inward and bend your elbow, holding the strap behind your back.
- Reach up your back with your left hand to grasp the strap, rolling your left shoulder back.

Adjust Your Feet

- Keep your feet touching or slightly wider than your hips.

Engage and Stretch

- Pull your hands in opposite directions using the strap.
- Sit tall and straight through your torso, neck, and head.

Breathe and Hold

- Inhale to lengthen your spine.
- Exhale to deepen the stretch, holding for 30 to 60 seconds with smooth, even breaths.

Release and Switch

- Release the strap and uncross your legs.
- Repeat on the opposite side, switching the strap to the left hand and reaching up with the right hand.

In this version, a strap is used to bridge the gap between the hands, which allows individuals with tight shoulders to achieve the full benefits of Cow Face Pose.

Camel Pose, or Ustrasana, is a backbend that involves kneeling and bending backward until your hands rest on your heels. This pose is known for its ability to improve flexibility, strength, and posture. It is often introduced in the middle or end of a yoga class when the body is adequately warmed up. Camel Pose offers numerous benefits, including opening the chest, lengthening the spine, strengthening the core, and challenging balance. Additionally, it can improve mental well-being by encouraging emotional openness and resilience.

Starting Position
- Kneel on the floor with your knees hip-width apart and your feet pointed behind you.
- If needed, place a blanket under your knees for cushioning and yoga blocks outside your ankles for modifications.

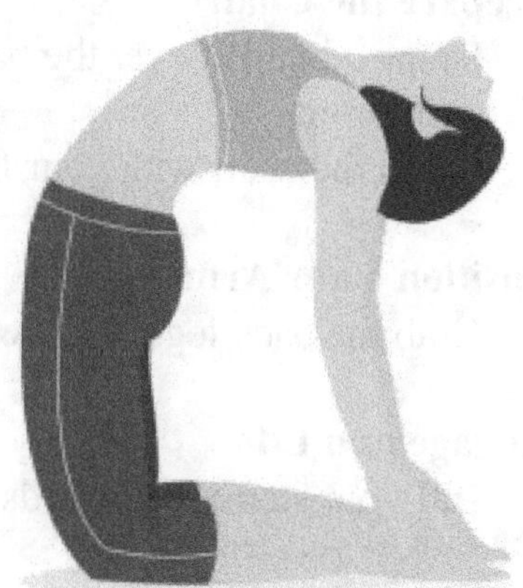

Engage Your Core
- Pull your belly button in and slightly tuck your tailbone to keep your pelvis in a neutral position.
- Place your hands on your waist, pulling your elbows back toward one another to knit your shoulder blades together.

Begin the Backbend
- Inhale deeply, lifting your breastbone toward the ceiling to initiate the backbend.
- Keep space in your lower back and use your upper back muscles to create a lift in your chest.

Pause and Adjust
- Pause here and, if comfortable, release your neck back in line with the spine.
- If you're ready, exhale and reach your hands back to grasp your heels or place your hands on the yoga blocks for support.

Deepen the Backbend
- Press into your shins and continue lifting your chest to deepen the backbend.
- Keep your inner thighs engaged and your shoulder blades firm against your back.

Hold the Pose
- Breathe deeply, holding the pose for a few breaths.
- Focus on maintaining a steady and comfortable breath.

Exit the Pose
- Inhale to lift your chest and come out of the backbend, restacking your spine.
- Sit back on your heels in Hero Pose (Virasana) and take a few breaths to rest.

Counterpose
- Counter the backbend by taking a Forward Fold (Uttanasana) to release any tension in your back.

Key Points

- Keep your core and inner thighs engaged to protect your lower back.
- Focus on lifting your chest and lengthening your spine to avoid compressing your lower back.
- Inhale to create space and lengthen, exhale to deepen the backbend.

Variation:

Camel Pose in a Chair

Prepare the Chair

- Drape a blanket over the back of the chair for added cushioning.
- Sit on the chair with your feet hip-distance apart.

Position Your Arms

- Grab the back legs of the chair with your arms stretched out.

Engage and Lift

- Lift your sternum upwards as you begin to arch your back.

Slide and Lean

- Slowly slide your hands down the back of the chair.
- For a more pronounced arch, press your upper shoulder blades onto the chair's back.

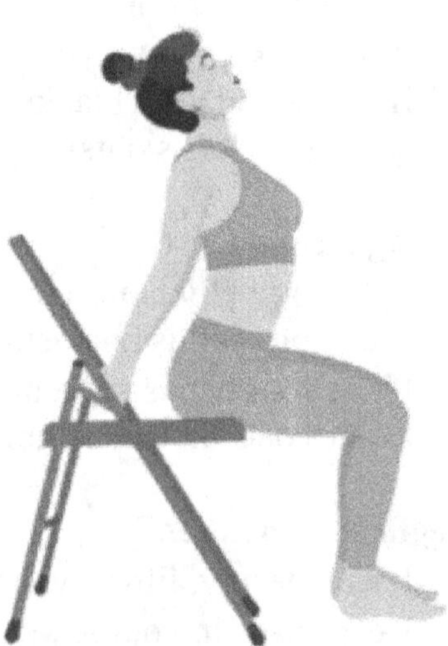

Adjust Your Head

- To keep your neck in a neutral position, tuck your chin in slightly toward your chest.

Hold and Breathe

- Hold the pose for a few breaths, focusing on lifting your chest and maintaining a gentle arch in your back.

Thread the Needle Pose (Parsva Balasana) is a gentle twist that provides a deep stretch to the shoulders, chest, and upper back. This pose is excellent for improving spinal mobility and relieving tension in the upper body. Practicing Thread the Needle helps to open the shoulders and can alleviate the stiffness that often comes from prolonged sitting or poor posture. It also encourages mindfulness and relaxation as it requires a steady breath and focus on the gentle twist.

Starting Position
- Begin in a neutral tabletop position with your hands and knees on your mat. Ensure your wrists are directly under your shoulders and your knees are under your hips.

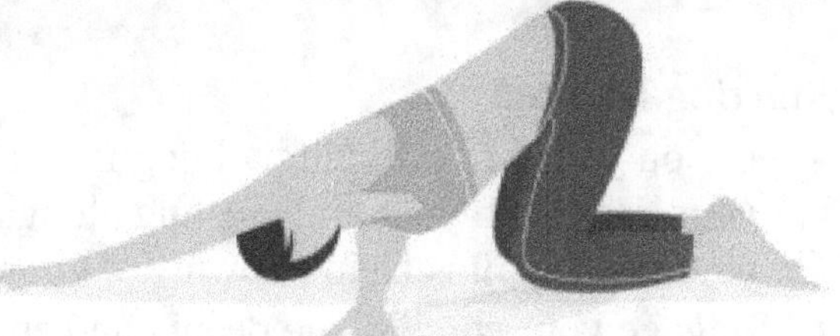

Thread the Needle
- Exhale and slide your right arm underneath your left arm, with your palm facing up. Lower your right shoulder and ear to the ground.

Position Legs and Feet
- Keep equal weight on your knees, with your feet straight out behind you. Your hips should remain lifted.

Hold the Pose
- Hold this position for 5-10 breaths, allowing each exhale to deepen the twist.

Return to Tabletop
- Inhale and press through your left hand to lift your torso back to the tabletop position.

Repeat on the Other Side
- Exhale and slide your left arm underneath your right arm, repeating the same steps on the opposite side.

Key Points
- Ensure your shoulders are aligned and avoid collapsing your chest.
- Keep your hips level and lifted to maintain balance.
- Use your breath to deepen the stretch gently, focusing on exhaling to enhance the twist.

Plow Pose, or Halasana, is a traditional yoga asana known for its numerous benefits, including stretching the shoulders, spine, and hamstrings while stimulating the thyroid gland and abdominal organs. This pose helps to calm the mind, reduce stress, and improve digestion. By reversing the blood flow, Plow Pose can also help relieve fatigue and rejuvenate the body and mind. Despite its restorative effects, it is important to practice this pose with care and proper alignment to avoid strain on the neck and spine.

Starting Position

- Lie on your back: Begin by lying flat on your back with your arms resting alongside your body, palms facing down.
- Engage your core: Inhale deeply and engage your core muscles to prepare for the lift.

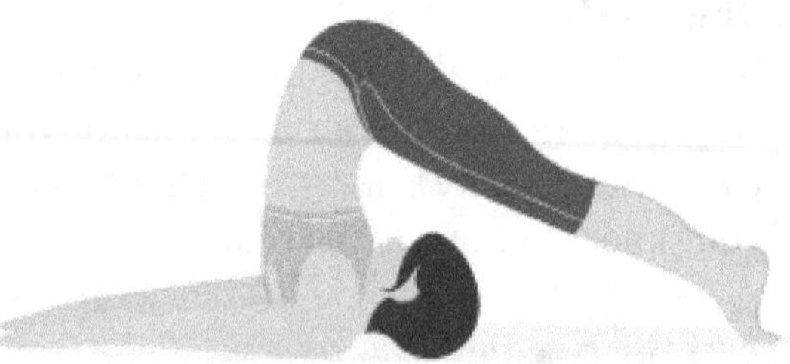

Lift Your Legs and Hips

- Raise your legs: On an exhale, lift your legs off the floor, bringing them perpendicular to the floor. Keep your legs straight and together.
- Lift your hips: Continue to lift your hips off the mat, bringing your legs up and over your head. Use your core strength to control the movement.

Extend Your Legs

- Reach your feet to the floor: Lower your legs and feet towards the floor behind your head. If your feet touch the floor, keep them flexed. If not, let them hover comfortably.
- Support your back: Place your hands on your lower back for support, with your elbows resting on the mat. Keep your upper arms firmly grounded to stabilize your pose.

Adjust and Hold the Pose

- Lengthen through your spine: Ensure that your spine is lengthening and your neck is relaxed. Avoid pressing your chin into your chest.
- Breathe deeply: Hold the pose for 5-10 breaths, breathing deeply and steadily. Focus on keeping your legs active and your core engaged.

Release the Pose

- Return your legs: To come out of the pose, gently bend your knees and slowly roll your spine back down to the mat, one vertebra at a time.
- Rest: Once you are lying flat on your back again, take a few deep breaths to relax and recover.

Key Points for Plow Pose (Halasana)

- Engage your core: Use your abdominal muscles to lift and control the movement of your legs and hips.
- Protect your neck: Avoid pressing your chin into your chest and ensure your neck is relaxed and free from strain.
- Breathe deeply: Maintain deep, steady breaths to help sustain the pose and keep your body relaxed.

Variation:

Starting Position

- Begin in Plow Pose: Start in Halasana with your legs extended over your head and your feet either on the floor or hovering above it.

Extend Your Legs Wider

- Open your legs: Gently separate your legs, bringing them wider apart. Keep your feet flexed and your legs active.
- Support your back: Keep your hands on your lower back for support, with your elbows grounded on the mat. Ensure your upper arms are stable.

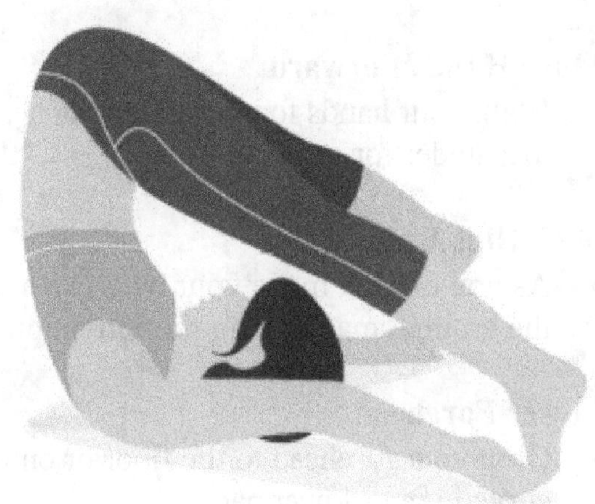

Adjust and Hold the Pose

- Lengthen through your spine: Maintain a long spine and relaxed neck. Avoid pressing your chin into your chest.
- Breathe deeply: Hold the wide-legged position for 5-10 breaths, focusing on deep, steady breathing. Feel the stretch in your inner thighs and hamstrings.

Release the Pose

- Bring your legs together: Slowly bring your legs back together over your head.
- Return your legs: Bend your knees slightly and gently roll your spine back down to the mat, one vertebra at a time.
- Rest: Once you are lying flat on your back again, take a few deep breaths to relax and recover.

Extended Puppy Pose (Uttana Shishosana) is a deeply restorative yoga pose that combines elements of a Child's Pose and a Downward-Facing Dog. This pose is excellent for stretching the spine, shoulders, and upper back. It helps to release tension in the entire back, making it beneficial for those who spend a lot of time sitting or have tightness in the upper body. Practicing Extended Puppy Pose can promote relaxation, reduce stress, and improve overall flexibility.

Starting Position

- Come onto all fours in a tabletop position with your shoulders above your wrists and hips above your knees.

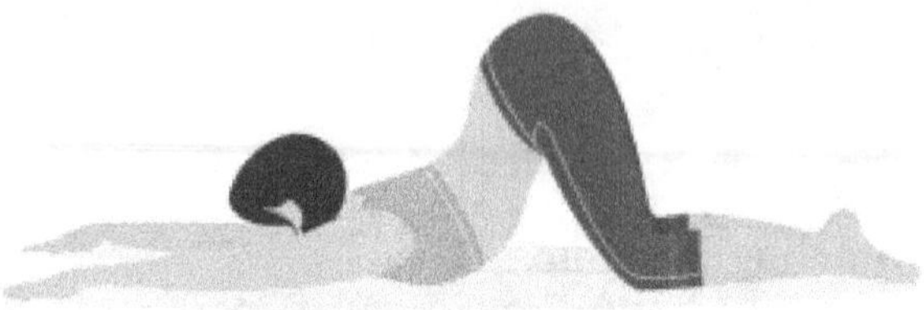

Move Hands Forward

- Walk your hands forward a few inches, ensuring your arms are active and engaged. Curl your toes under for stability.

Shift Hips Back

- As you exhale, move your buttocks halfway back toward your heels. Keep your elbows off the ground, maintaining the activation in your arms.

Lower Forehead

- Drop your forehead to the floor or onto a blanket. Let your neck relax and maintain a slight curve in your lower back.

Stretch and Breathe

- Press your hands down firmly and stretch through your arms while pulling your hips back toward your heels. Breathe deeply into your back, feeling the spine lengthen in both directions.

Hold the Pose

- Hold for 30 seconds to a minute, breathing deeply and allowing your body to relax into the stretch.

Release

- To come out of the pose, exhale and release your buttocks down onto your heels, returning to a seated position.

Key Points

- Keep your arms active and engaged to enhance the stretch in your shoulders and upper back.
- Ensure your hips remain lifted to maintain the alignment and effectiveness of the stretch.
- Focus on deep, steady breaths to help lengthen the spine and deepen the stretch.

Variation:

Starting Position
- Begin in a tabletop position with shoulders above wrists and hips above knees.

Use Blocks
- Place yoga blocks under your forearms for additional support and to enhance the stretch.

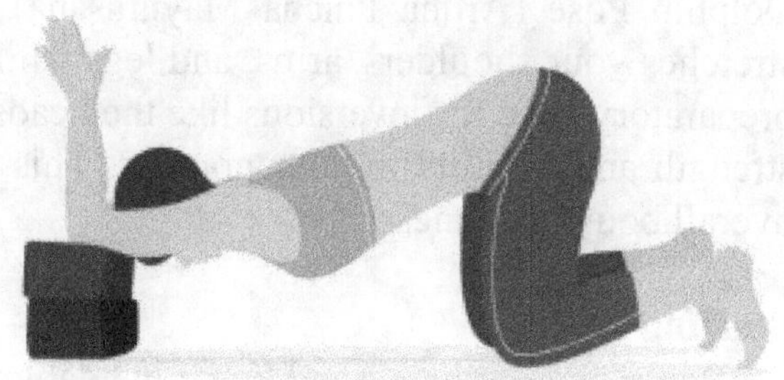

Move Hands Forward
- Walk your hands forward, keeping your forearms on the blocks and arms active.

Shift Hips Back
- Exhale and move your buttocks halfway back toward your heels.

Lower Forehead
- Drop your forehead to the floor or onto a blanket.

Stretch and Breathe
- Press your forearms into the blocks, stretching through your arms and pulling your hips back.

Hold the Pose
- Hold for 30 seconds to a minute, focusing on your breath and deepening the stretch.

Release
- Exhale and release your buttocks down onto your heels, then remove the blocks and return to a seated position.

Dolphin Pose (Ardha Pincha Mayurasana) is an excellent yoga posture that strengthens and stretches your shoulders, arms, and legs while also improving balance and flexibility. It's a great preparatory pose for inversions like the headstand and forearm stand, making it ideal for building strength and stability in your practice. This pose also engages your core muscles and enhances overall body awareness.

Starting Position
- Begin on your hands and knees in a tabletop position.
- Align your wrists under your shoulders and your knees under your hips.

Position Your Arms
- Lower your forearms to the floor, keeping your elbows shoulder-width apart.
- Interlace your fingers or place your palms flat on the ground.

Lift Your Hips
- Tuck your toes under and, on an exhale, lift your knees off the floor.
- Straighten your legs as much as possible, lifting your hips towards the ceiling.
- Keep your head between your upper arms without letting it hang or pressing it into the ground.

Engage Your Shoulders and Core
- Press firmly into your forearms and wrists to lift and open your shoulders.
- Engage your core muscles to stabilize your body and prevent your lower back from arching excessively.

Adjust Your Feet
- Walk your feet slightly closer to your hands if needed, maintaining the lift in your hips.
- Keep your feet hip-width apart and press your heels towards the floor.

Hold and Breathe
- Stay in the pose for 5-10 breaths, focusing on deep, steady breathing.
- Lengthen your spine and keep your shoulders engaged.

Release
- To come out of the pose, gently lower your knees back to the floor and return to the tabletop position.

Key Points
- Keep your forearms firmly on the ground and lift through your shoulders.
- Focus on lifting your hips towards the ceiling to create length in your spine.
- Maintain deep, steady breaths throughout the pose to enhance stability and relaxation.

Starting Position
- Begin in Dolphin Pose, with your forearms on the ground and hips lifted high.

Lift One Leg
- Inhale deeply and, on your exhale, lift your right leg towards the ceiling.
- Keep your hips level and your lifted leg straight, engaging your core for stability.

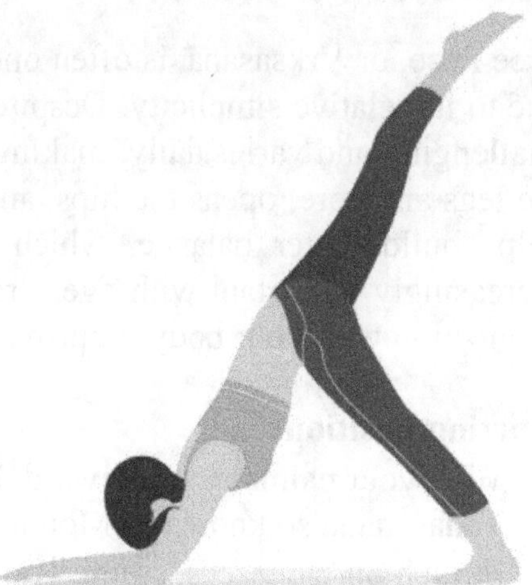

Maintain Alignment
- Press firmly into your forearms and keep your shoulders engaged.
- Ensure your head stays between your upper arms and doesn't drop or press into the ground.

Adjust Your Supporting Leg
- Keep your left foot firmly grounded, pressing the heel towards the floor.
- Maintain a straight line from your lifted foot through your supporting leg and torso.

Hold and Breathe
- Hold the pose for 3-5 breaths, keeping your lifted leg active and engaged.
- Focus on deep, steady breathing to maintain balance and stability.

Switch Sides
- On an exhale, lower your right leg back to the floor and return to Dolphin Pose.
- Repeat the same steps with your left leg lifted.

Release
- To come out of the pose, gently lower both knees to the floor and return to the tabletop position.

Tree Pose (Vrksasana)

Tree Pose, or Vrksasana, is often one of the first standing balance poses taught to yoga beginners due to its relative simplicity. Despite its straightforward appearance, balancing on one leg can be challenging and varies daily, making it a humbling and insightful practice. Tree Pose strengthens the legs and core, opens the hips, and stretches the inner thigh and groin muscles. This pose also helps build better balance, which is beneficial for various physical activities and becomes increasingly important with age. Practicing Tree Pose encourages a sense of groundedness and connection with your body, improving posture, alignment, and confidence.

Starting Position
- With your palms facing inward, in the Anjali Mudra, stand tall in Tadasana, also known as Mountain Pose.
- Stretch out your toes, stomp your feet firmly on the mat, and tense your leg muscles.

Shift Your Weight
- As you lift your left foot off the floor, start shifting your weight onto your right foot.
- Do not lock your knee and keep a straight right leg.

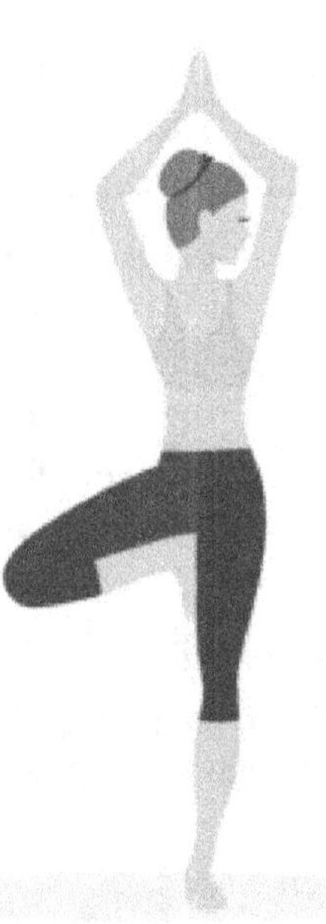

Position Your Foot
- Bend your left knee and place your left foot on your inner right leg or shin.
- You should not put your foot on your knee.

Engage and Align
- Press your left foot and right leg into each other to create stability.
- Ensure your pelvis is level and square to the front.

Arm Position
- When stable, perform Anjali Mudra at your heart or spread your arms upwards like branches reaching for the sun.

Focus and Breathe
- Focus your gaze (Drishti) on a fixed point to help maintain balance.
- Lift your chest and exhale as you bring your shoulder blades down your back.
- Hold for several breaths, maintaining steady and even breathing.

Release the Pose
- Lower your left foot to the floor and return to Mountain Pose.
- Repeat on the other side, shifting your weight into your left foot and lifting your right foot.

Key Points
- Focus on pressing your foot into your thigh and your thigh back into your foot to maintain stability.
- Keep your pelvis level and squared to the front to avoid hip misalignment.

Variation

Tree Pose Hand on the Wall (Vrksasana)

Starting Position
- Stand next to a wall with your left side facing it.
- Place your left hand on the wall for support.

Shift Your Weight
- Instead of keeping your left foot flat on the ground, transfer your weight to your right foot.
- Do not lock your knee, but do maintain a straight right leg.

Position Your Foot
- Bend your left knee and place your left foot on your inner right leg or shin.
- Avoid placing your foot squarely on your kneecap.

Engage and Align
- Press your left foot and right leg into each other to create stability.
- Ensure your pelvis is level and square to the front.

Use the Wall for Support
- Keep your left hand on the wall to help maintain balance.
- If comfortable, you can gradually reduce the pressure of your hand on the wall or try lifting it slightly off for brief moments.

Arm Position
- Place your right hand into Anjali Mudra at your heart or stretch your right arm overhead like a tree branch reaching into the sun.

Focus and Breathe
- Focus your gaze (Drishti) on a fixed point to help maintain balance.
- Breathe in deeply while raising your chest, and then let go as you lower your shoulders back.
- Hold for several breaths, maintaining steady and even breathing.

Lower your left foot to the floor and return to Mountain Pose.
Repeat on the other side, turning to face the wall with your right hand to provide support and lift your right foot.

The Standing Lunge Stretch is an excellent exercise for not only strengthening the legs and glutes but also stretching the hip flexors, groin, and inner thighs. This versatile stretch can enhance flexibility and mobility in the lower body, making it an essential component of any fitness routine. Strengthen your lower body and lessen the likelihood of injury by including this stretch in your routine.

Starting Position
- Maintain a neutral stance with your arms resting at your sides and your feet spaced hip-width apart.

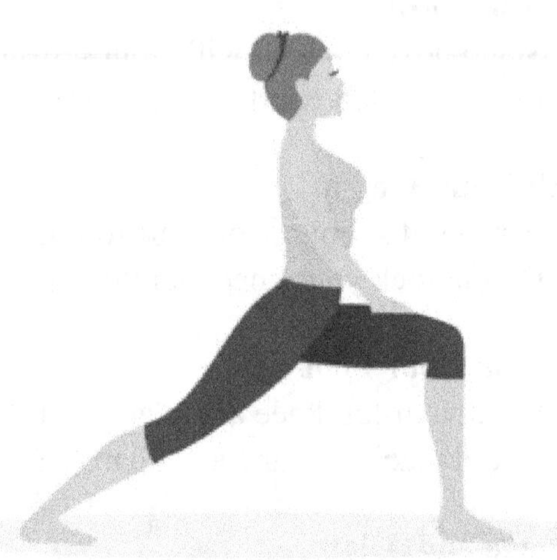

Step Forward
- Make a split stance by stepping forward with your right foot.
- Keep your left leg extended straight back behind you.

Lower Your Body
- Place your hands on your hips or on your forward knee for support.
- Lower your right knee to 90 degrees, directly above your ankle.
- Your left leg should remain extended and straight, with your heel lifted off the ground.

Hold the Stretch
- Inhale deeply to lengthen your spine.
- Feel the hip flexors, groin, and inner thighs stretch as you exhale.
- While holding the stretch, breathe deeply and evenly for 20-30 seconds.

Release and Switch Sides
- Inhale and step back to the starting position.
- Repeat the stretch on the other side by stepping forward with your left foot and lowering your left knee to 90 degrees.

Key Points
- Avoid straining your front knee by placing it directly over your ankle.
- Balance yourself and protect your lower back by keeping your abs tight.
- Use your breath to deepen the stretch and maintain relaxation throughout the pose.

Variation:

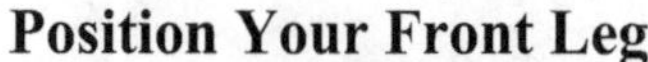

Starting Position
- Kneel on a yoga mat or exercise mat with both knees.
- Sit back so your bottom rests on your heels, and the balls of your feet press firmly against the mat.

Lean Forward
- Maintaining a distance of shoulder-width between your hands, lean forward and bring your palms down to the mat.
- Slightly bend your elbows to prevent them from locking.

Position Your Front Leg
- Make a right angle by bringing your left knee forward between your arms and placing your left foot flat on the mat ahead of you.

Adjust Your Upper Body
- Straighten your upper body and place both hands on your left knee for support and balance.

Extend Your Back Leg
- Extend your right leg behind you, pressing your right knee into the mat.
- Rest the top of your right foot on the mat.

Deepen the Stretch
- Inhale deeply to lengthen your spine.
- Exhale and lean forward slightly to deepen the stretch in your right hip flexor.
- Hold the stretch for 20–30 seconds, inhaling deeply and evenly.

Release and Switch Sides
- Inhale and return to the starting position.
- Exhale and repeat the stretch on the opposite side by bringing your right knee forward and extending your left leg behind you.

The Bound Angle Pose, which is also referred to as Baddha Konasana or Cobbler's Pose, is a fundamental yoga position that promotes hip opening and stretches the muscles that are located within the inner thighs. This seemingly basic stance also helps to strengthen your core and improve your posture by working your back muscles and stretching your spine. While it may appear straightforward, holding Bound Angle Pose for an extended period can be challenging as it requires sustained effort from the back, hip, thigh, and hamstring muscles. This pose enhances postural and body awareness, making it beneficial for recovery after physical activities like running and for those who spend a lot of time sitting.

Starting Position
- Begin in Staff Pose (Dandasana) with your legs extended straight in front of you.
- Place your weight squarely on your sitting bones rather than behind them.

Bend Your Knees
- Get down on all fours and spread your legs wide.
- Bring your heel to a point where it is comfortable with your pelvis, and bring the soles of your feet together.

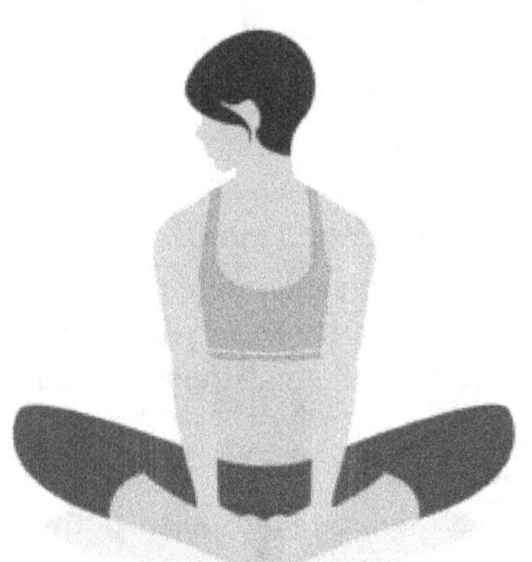

Position Your Feet
- Use your hands to open your feet as if you were opening the pages of a book.
- Keep the outer edges of your feet pressed together.

Engage and Lift
- For a chest raise, press your shoulder blades into your upper back.
- Clasp your ankles or feet to help you find lift along your torso.

Hold the Pose
- Inhale deeply to lengthen your spine.
- Exhale and gently press your knees towards the floor without forcing.
- Hold the pose for several breaths, maintaining a long spine and open chest.

To exit, gently release your feet and extend your legs back into Staff Pose.

Key Points
- Keep your spine long and avoid rounding your back.
- Press your knees towards the floor without forcing, allowing a gentle stretch.
- Engage your core to support your back and maintain an upright posture.

Variation:

Starting Position
- Begin in Staff Pose (Dandasana) with your legs extended straight in front of you.
- Place your weight squarely on your sitting bones rather than behind them.

Bend Your Knees
- Get down on all fours and spread your legs wide.
- Bring your heel to a point where it is comfortable with your pelvis, and bring the soles of your feet together.

Position Your Feet
- Use your hands to open your feet as if you were opening the pages of a book.
- Keep the outer edges of your feet pressed together.

Add Props
- If your knees remain far from the ground, place yoga blocks under your knees for support.
- Alternatively, slide-folded or rolled blankets under your shins and thighs to provide cushioning and support.

Engage and Lift
- For a chest raise, press your shoulder blades into your upper back.
- Clasp your ankles or feet to help you find lift along your torso.

Hold the Pose
- Inhale deeply to lengthen your spine.
- Exhale and gently press your knees towards the props, allowing a gentle stretch without forcing.
- Hold the pose for several breaths, maintaining a long spine and open chest.

To exit, gently release your feet and extend your legs back into Staff Pose.

Pigeon Pose, or Eka Pada Rajakapotasana, is an essential yoga pose that deeply opens the hips, enhancing flexibility and circulation in the lower body. Tight hips can restrict your range of motion and cause discomfort, making this pose particularly beneficial. Pigeon Pose stretches the thighs, groin, back, piriformis, and psoas muscles, addressing both external rotation and hip flexor lengthening. Practicing this pose with mindful attention to alignment can promote a sense of calm and clarity while significantly improving overall mobility and comfort in both seated postures and daily activities.

Starting Position
- Begin in Downward Facing Dog.
- Step into a Down Dog Split with your right leg up.

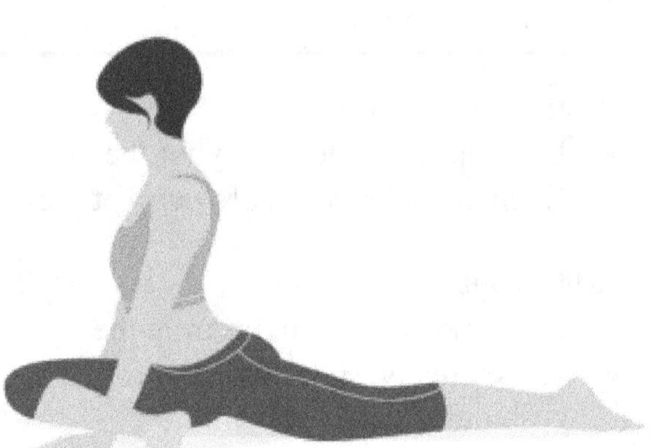

Bring the Knee Forward
- As you would step into a lunge, bend your right knee and bring it forward.
- Place your right knee on the floor outside your right hand.
- If you're flexible enough, you can angle your right shin toward your left hip, or you can bring it parallel to the mat.

Position the Back Leg
- Release your left knee to the mat.
- Extend your left leg straight back, with the top of your thigh resting on the floor.
- Look back to ensure your left foot is pointing straight back.

Square the Hips
- Square your hips toward the front of your mat.
- Use padding under your right hip if necessary to make the pose more comfortable.

Forward Bend (Optional)
- If stable, bring your torso down into a forward bend over your right leg.
- Keep your hips square and distribute weight equally on both sides.
- Reach your forehead toward the floor and breathe deeply.

Hold the Pose
- Inhale deeply to lengthen your spine.
- Exhale and sink deeper into the stretch, holding the pose for several breaths.

Release the Pose
- Step back into Downward Facing Dog and curl your left toes to release.
- Repeat the pose on the other side.

Key Points
- Ensure your hips are squared to the front to avoid imbalance and strain.
- Use blankets or blocks under your hip or back knee for additional support and comfort.
- Focus on deep, steady breaths to help release tension and deepen the stretch.

Variations:

Starting Position
- Sit on a chair: Sit comfortably on a chair with your feet flat on the floor, hip-width apart. Keep your spine straight and shoulders relaxed.

Cross Your Leg
- Lift your right leg: Lift your right leg and place your right ankle on your left thigh, just above the knee. Your right foot should be flexed to protect your knee joint.

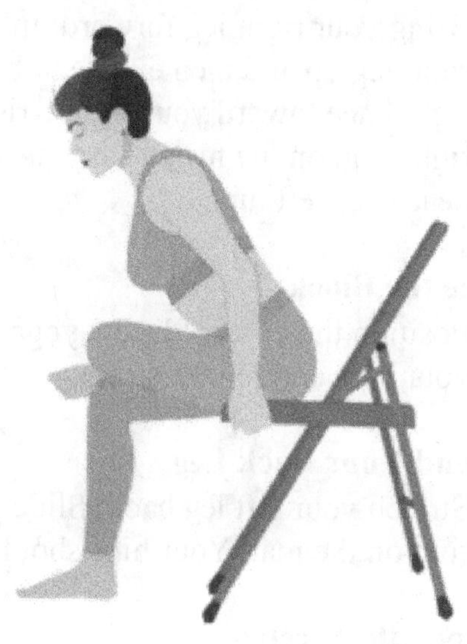

Adjust Your Position
- Align your posture: Sit up straight, ensuring that your spine is lengthened and your shoulders are relaxed. Your right knee should be pointing out to the side.
- Breathe deeply: Take a deep breath in and exhale slowly, allowing your body to settle into the position.

Deepen the Stretch
- Lean forward: On an exhale, gently lean forward from your hips, keeping your spine straight. Place your hands on your right shin or thigh for support.
- Hold the pose: Hold this position for 5-10 breaths, feeling the stretch in your right hip and glute. Breathe deeply and steadily.

Release the Pose
- Return to sitting upright: Inhale and slowly come back to an upright position.
- Switch sides: Release your right leg and place your foot back on the floor. Repeat the pose on the other side with your left leg.

Starting Position

- Begin in Downward-Facing Dog: Start in
  Adho Mukha Svanasana (Downward-Facing
  Dog) with your hands shoulder-width apart
  and your feet hip-width apart.

Step Your Leg Forward

- Bring your right leg forward: Inhale, lift your
  right leg up and then exhale to bring your
  right knee toward your right wrist. Place your
  right shin on the mat, with your right foot
  near your left hip.

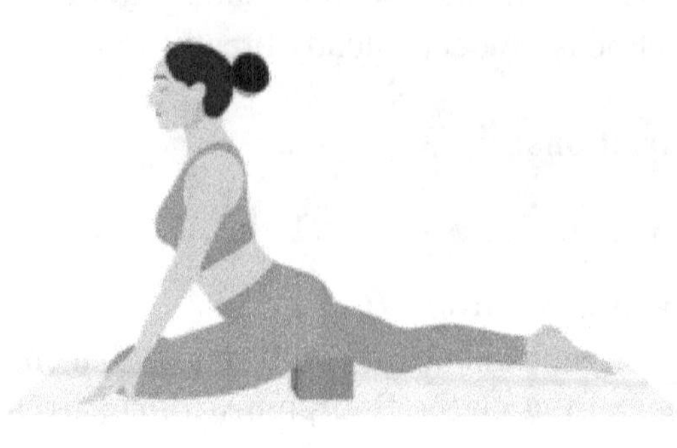

Place the Block

- Position the block: Place a yoga block under your right hip for support. This helps to level
  your hips and reduce strain.

Extend Your Back Leg

- Stretch your left leg back: Slide your left leg back, keeping it straight with the top of your
  foot on the mat. Your hips should be squared to the front of the mat.

Deepen the Stretch

- Lower your torso: On an exhale, slowly lower your torso over your right shin. You can place
  your forearms on the mat or stack your hands and rest your forehead on them.
- Hold the pose: Stay here for 5-10 breaths, feeling the stretch in your hips and glutes. Ensure
  your left leg remains active and your hips are level.

Release the Pose

- Come back to Downward-Facing Dog: Inhale to lift your torso and press your hands into the
  mat. Exhale to step back into Downward-Facing Dog.
- Switch sides: Repeat the pose on the other side with your left leg forward.

One-Legged Pigeon Pose, or Eka Pada Rajakapotasana, is a powerful hip opener that stretches the hip flexors and the glutes. It is known for its deep release and is often used in yoga sequences to increase flexibility in the hips and relieve tension in the lower back. This pose also encourages a forward fold, which can be calming for the mind and body, helping to reduce stress and anxiety.

Starting Position

- Begin in Downward-Facing Dog: Start on your hands and knees in a tabletop position, then lift your hips and straighten your legs to come into Downward-Facing Dog.
- Inhale deeply: Take a deep breath in, preparing to move your leg.

Bring Your Leg Forward

- Step forward: On an exhale, bring your right knee forward towards your right wrist. Your right ankle should be near your left wrist, with your shin resting on the floor.
- Extend your left leg: Slide your left leg straight back behind you, ensuring your hips remain square to the front of your mat.

Align Your Hips

- Square your hips: Keep your hips level and squared to the front of your mat. If needed, place a folded blanket or a block under your right hip to maintain balance and alignment.
- Engage your legs: Actively press your back leg into the floor, extending through your left toes.

Lower Your Torso

- Inhale and lengthen: Lengthen your spine, reaching the crown of your head up.
- Exhale and fold: As you exhale, walk your hands forward and lower your torso over your right shin, resting your forehead on the mat, a block, or your forearms.

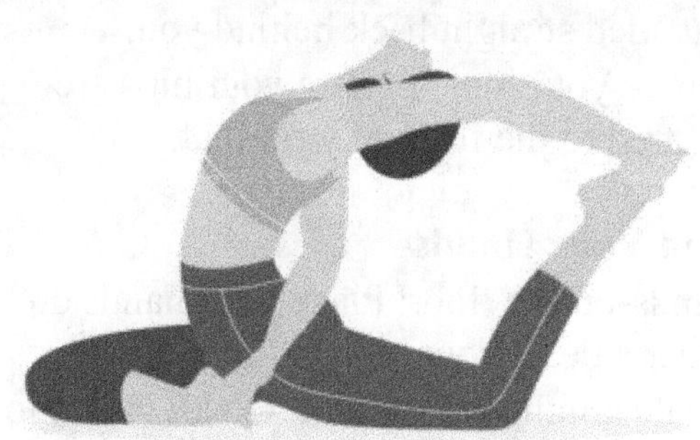

Hold the Pose

- Breathe deeply: Stay in the pose for 5-10 deep breaths, relaxing into the stretch with each exhale.
- Relax your body: Allow your hips to release and your body to sink deeper into the pose with each breath.

Release the Pose

- Walk your hands back: On an inhale, walk your hands back towards your body, lifting your torso upright.
- Return to Downward-Facing Dog: Tuck your left toes under, lift your hips, and step back to Downward-Facing Dog. Repeat on the other side.

Key Points

- Keep your hips square and level to avoid straining the lower back.
- Use props like blocks or blankets to support your hips and maintain proper alignment.
- Focus on deep, steady breaths to help release tension and deepen the stretch.

Starting Position

- Begin in Pigeon Pose: Start in the standard Pigeon Pose (Eka Pada Rajakapotasana) with your right knee bent and your right shin on the floor while your left leg is extended straight back behind you.
- Square your hips: Ensure your hips are squared to the front of your mat.

Position Your Hands

- Hands-on the floor: Place your hands on either side of your hips for support.
- Inhale and lift your chest: On an inhalation, lift your torso and lengthen your spine, pressing your hands into the floor.

Bend Your Back Leg

- Reach for your back foot: Bend your left knee and reach your left hand back to grasp your left foot or ankle. If this is challenging, use a yoga strap around your foot.
- Lift through your chest: Keep your chest lifted and your spine long as you draw your left foot closer to your head.

Extend Your Other Arm

- Reach up and back: Extend your right arm up towards the ceiling and then back to grasp your left foot, joining your hands in a clasp if possible.
- Open your chest: Press your shoulder blades together and open your chest towards the ceiling.

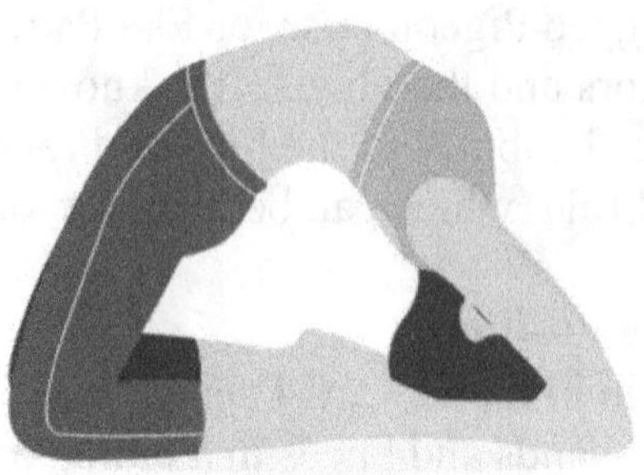

Deepen the Pose

- Backbend and lengthen: Continue to lift through your chest and lengthen your spine, deepening the backbend. Ensure you are not compressing your lower back.
- Engage your core: Maintain engagement through your core to support your lower back and hips.

Hold the Pose

- Breathe deeply: Stay in the pose for 3-5 deep breaths, maintaining the lift and openness in your chest and the length of your spine.

Release the Pose

- Slowly release your foot: Gently release your back foot and bring your hands back to the floor.
- Return to Pigeon Pose: Straighten your back leg and return to the standard Pigeon Pose before switching sides.

Key Points

- Focus on lifting and opening your chest to deepen the backbend.
- Keep your hips squared to the front of your mat to ensure proper alignment.
- Engage your core muscles to support your lower back and maintain stability.

Reclined Big Toe Pose, or Supta Padangusthasana, is a highly effective yoga posture that deeply stretches the hips, thighs, hamstrings, groins, and calves. This pose not only enhances flexibility but also helps in relieving tension and tightness in the lower body. Practicing this pose regularly can improve your range of motion and promote relaxation, making it a valuable addition to any yoga routine.

Starting Position
- Begin in a supine position (lying on your back) with your legs together and feet flexed, similar to Tadasana (Mountain Pose).

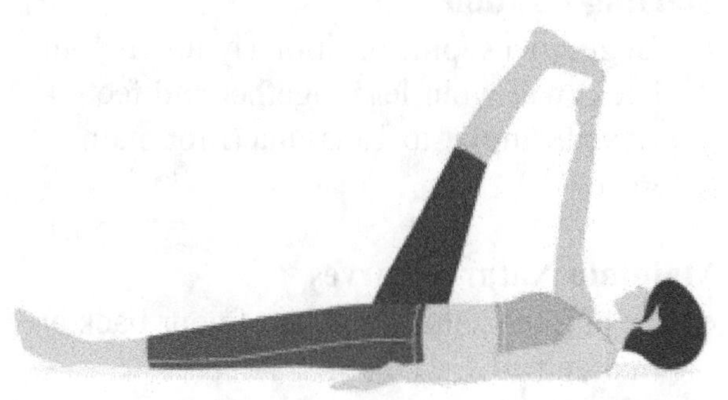

Maintain Natural Curves
- Ensure the natural curves of your back are maintained.
- Your hand should fit behind your neck and under your small back without flattening your lower back.

Bend and Lift
- Bend your right knee and bring it up to your chest without bending your lower back.
- Clasp your hands together at the knee and grasp your thigh.
- Keep your left leg straight and engaged while anchoring it to the mat.

Loop Your Toe
- Loop your big toe with the first two fingers of your right hand.
- While maintaining a strong and engaged core in both legs, start to straighten your right leg toward the ceiling.

Adjust and Stretch
- Your ability to bring your leg in closer to your chest while maintaining a straight or slightly bent leg depends on how flexible your hamstrings are.
- To lengthen your spine, take a long breath in and then exhale to make the stretch even deeper.

Hold the Pose
- Hold this pose for 5 breaths, maintaining steady and even breathing.
- Ensure both legs remain engaged and your back stays in its natural curve.

Release and Switch Sides
- Let your right leg fall slowly.
- Repeat the pose on the opposite side by bending your left knee and lifting it toward your chest.

Key Points

- Ensure your back maintains its natural curves, avoiding flattening the lower back.
- Keep the muscles in both legs strong and engaged throughout the pose.
- Use deep, steady breaths to lengthen the spine and deepen the stretch.

Variation:

Reclined Big Toe Pose with a Strap (Supta Padangusthasana Variation)

Starting Position

- Begin in a supine position (lying on your back) with your legs together and feet flexed, similar to Tadasana (Mountain Pose).

Maintain Natural Curves

- Ensure the natural curves of your back are maintained.
- Your hand should fit behind your neck and under your small back without flattening your lower back.

Bend and Lift

- Bend your right knee and lift it to your chest without slouching.
- Hold your thigh with both hands clasped near your knee.
- Keep your left leg straight and engaged while anchoring it to the mat.

Loop the Strap

- Loop a yoga strap around the sole of your right foot, wherever it is comfortable.
- Hold the strap with both hands, extending your arms without straining.

Straighten the Leg

- Use the strap to straighten your right leg toward the ceiling.
- Maintain a strong and engaged quadriceps.

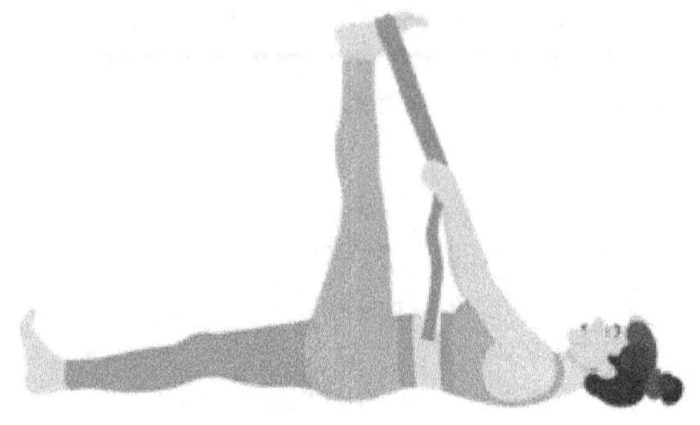

Adjust and Stretch

- Put your right leg closer to the floor or slightly bend your knee if you have knee discomfort or sharpness.
- You should feel sensations in the center of your hamstring or muscle belly, not the joint.
- To lengthen your spine, take a long breath in and then exhale to make the stretch even deeper.

Hold the Pose

- Hold this pose for 5 breaths, maintaining steady and even breathing.
- Ensure both legs remain engaged and your back stays in its natural curve.

Release and Switch Sides

- Slowly release the strap and lower your right leg to the floor.
- Repeat the pose on the opposite side by bending your left knee and lifting it toward your chest, then looping the strap around your left foot.

Happy Baby Pose, or Ananda Balasana, is a gentle yet effective yoga posture that stretches, strengthens, and relaxes various areas of your body. This pose mimics the position of a happy baby on its back and is both restful and restorative. It offers a deep stretch for the inner thighs, groins, hips, hamstrings, and even the shoulders and chest. Practicing Happy Baby Pose can decompress the sacroiliac (SI) joints, open the hips, release tension from the spine and sacrum, and calm the mind, reducing stress and fatigue. This pose is often used at the beginning of a yoga session to warm up the body or at the end to wind down and relax.

Starting Position
- Lie flat on your back on a comfortable surface, such as a yoga mat.
- Gently exhale and bring your knees toward your chest.

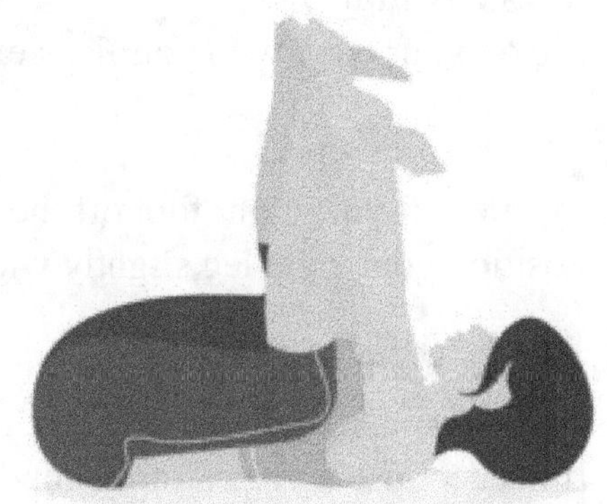

Open Your Knees
- Open your knees wider than your body and bring them to your armpits.
- Keep your lower back pressed to the ground.

Position Your Ankles and Shins
- Each ankle should be directly over its knee, with shins perpendicular to the floor.
- To activate the muscles in your legs, bend at the ankles.

Grip Your Feet
- Extend your arms alongside your inner thighs and grab the outer edges of your feet.
- If you can't reach your feet, tie a yoga strap around each other and grip your big toes with your index and middle fingers.

Create Counterpressure
- Gently push your feet into your hands (or the straps) while simultaneously pulling down with your hands to create counterpressure.
- Bring the soles of your feet up so they face the ceiling, keeping your knees bent and forming a right angle with each leg.

Maintain Alignment and Relax
- Ensure your tailbone and spine remain on the floor; do not lift your hips off the mat.
- Let your head lie softly on the mat as you keep your shoulders and neck relaxed.
- Relax here for up to one minute, keeping your breaths deep and steady.

Release the Pose
- Gently let go of your feet and bring your knees back together.
- Briefly hug your knees to your chest before extending your legs back to the starting position.
- Reach your arms overhead for a full-body stretch.

Key Points
- Keep your tailbone and spine on the floor; avoid lifting your hips off the mat.
- Engage your leg muscles by flexing your feet and creating counterpressure with your hands.
- To stretch and relax, relax your neck and shoulders and breathe deeply.

Variation:

Starting Position
- Lie on your back with your legs extended and arms by your sides.

Lift One Leg
- Exhale, lift your right foot off the mat, bend your knee, and bring it toward your belly.
- Position your right leg slightly wider than your torso, with the knee toward your armpit.

Grip Your Foot
- Grip the outside of your right foot with your right hand.
- If needed, use a yoga strap around your foot.

Create Counterpressure
- Gently push your foot into your hand (or strap) and pull down with your hand.
- Keep your left leg extended and pressed into the mat.

Maintain Alignment and Relax
- Ensure your lower back and sacrum stay on the floor.
- Relax your neck and shoulders, holding for several breaths.

Release and Switch Sides
- Release your right foot and extend your leg back.
- Repeat on the left side.

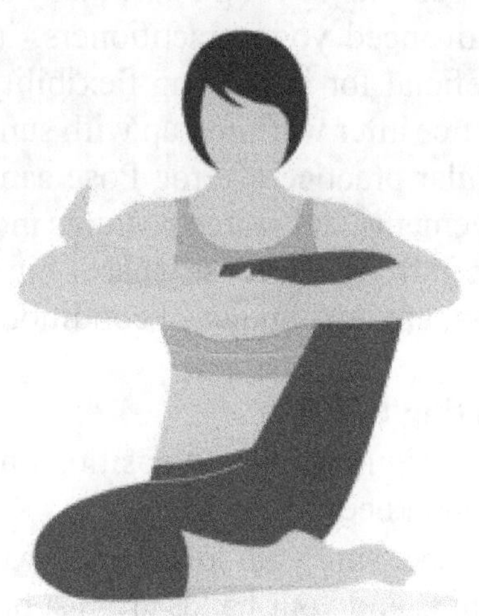

Starting Position

- Sit in a comfortable seat: Begin in a seated position, preferably in Dandasana (Staff Pose), with your legs extended straight in front of you and your back straight.

Lift and Cross Your Leg

- Bend your right knee: Bend your right knee and bring it toward your chest.
- Lift your right foot: Use both hands to lift your right foot and place it in the crease of your left elbow.
- Cradle your leg: Wrap your right arm around the outside of your right knee, holding your right leg as if you are cradling a baby.

Position Your Hands

- Interlace your fingers: Interlace your fingers around your right shin or hold onto your right foot and knee, creating a secure cradle for your leg.
- Sit up tall: Lengthen your spine and sit up tall, engaging your core muscles to maintain balance.

Deepen the Stretch

- Rock gently: Gently rock your leg back and forth, side to side, like you are soothing a baby. This motion helps to open your hip and stretch your glute muscles.
- Breathe deeply: Take deep breaths in and out, using your breath to help you relax and deepen the stretch.

Switch Sides

- Release the leg: Gently release your right leg and extend it back to the starting position.
- Repeat on the other side: Bend your left knee, lift your left foot, and cradle your left leg in the same way.

The benefits of Frog Pose, also called Mandukasana, which are well-known among intermediate to advanced yoga practitioners, include opening the hips and groins. This pose is particularly beneficial for improving flexibility, circulation, and posture. It's an excellent addition to a yoga practice after warming up with sun salutations and lunges, preparing your hips for a deeper stretch. Regular practice of Frog Pose can enhance mobility and flexibility in the hips, making everyday movements and seated postures more comfortable. Those who sit for long periods of time will also benefit from it because it eases hip and lower back pain. Additionally, Frog Pose may help manage stress, anxiety, and even conditions like diabetes by regulating blood sugar levels.

Starting Position

- Begin in a tabletop position on your hands and knees.
- Make sure your knees are lower than your hips and your hands are just beneath your shoulders.
- Breathe deeply for three to five breaths to center yourself.

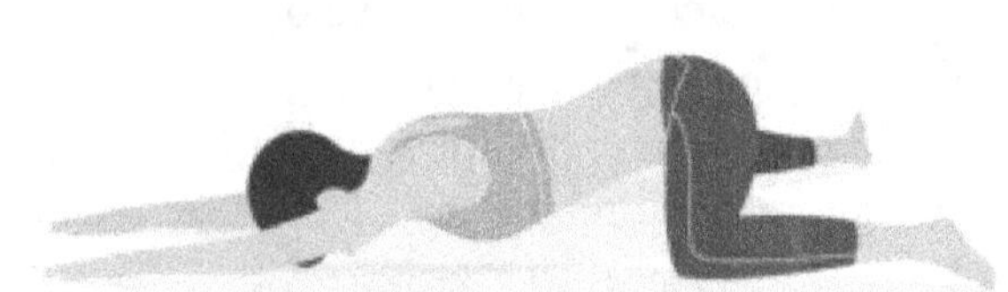

Move Your Knees Outward

- Inhale deeply, then exhale as you slowly move your right and left knees outward to the sides.
- Stop and hold the position, breathing deeply whenever you feel the stretch.

Adjust Your Feet and Ankles

- Turn your feet outward, flexing your ankles so that the inner feet, inner ankles, and inner knees touch the floor.
- If needed, place a blanket under your ankles for cushioning.

Lower to Your Forearms

- Slowly lower down to your forearms, keeping your palms flat on the floor or pressing them together.
- If this is too intense, stay on your palms or place your forearms on blocks.

Hold the Pose

- Stay in this position for five to ten breaths or as long as it is comfortable.
- Ensure your breathing remains deep and steady; adjust if your breathing becomes short or forced.

Release the Pose

- To release, slowly slide your knees closer together and return to the tabletop position.
- Alternatively, slide your feet together and press your hips back into a wide-kneed variation of Child's Pose.

Key Points

- Keep your knees aligned with your hips and ensure they are well-cushioned.
- Maintain deep, steady breaths to gauge the appropriateness of the stretch.
- Utilize blankets or blocks to support your knees and forearms, ensuring comfort and proper alignment.

Garland Pose, or Malasana, is a deep squat that opens the hips and groin, counterbalancing the tightness often developed from prolonged sitting. This pose stretches and strengthens the feet and ankles while promoting long-term mobility and pain prevention. While squatting is a natural resting position in many cultures, it can be uncomfortable for those unaccustomed to it. Using props initially can help ease into the pose, allowing for gradual adaptation and improvement in flexibility and comfort.

Starting Position
- Stand with your feet about mat-width apart.
- Turn your toes out slightly but avoid overdoing it.

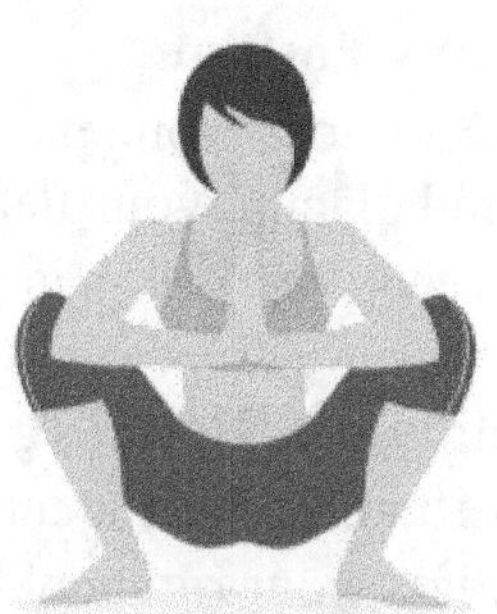

Lower into the Squat
- Bend your knees and lower your buttocks toward the floor into a squat.
- Keep your feet as parallel as possible over time, working toward a more neutral position.

Position Your Arms
- Bring your upper arms inside your knees.
- In the Anjali Mudra (prayer pose), with your palms facing each other and your elbows bent, locate the center of your heart.

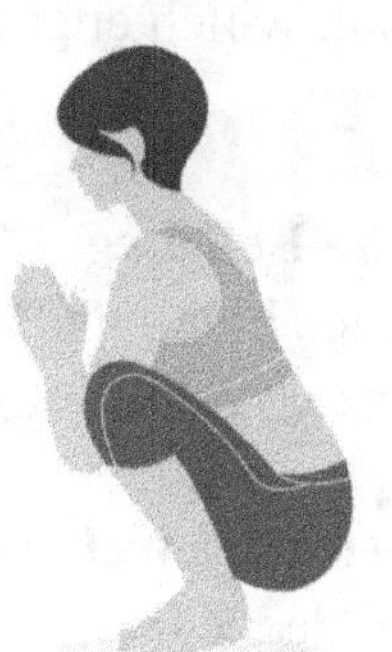

Engage and Lift
- Press your thumbs against your sternum to help lift your chest.
- Hold the position by pressing your upper arms into your thighs and vice versa.

Maintain Alignment
- Keep your spine straight and your buttocks moving toward the floor.
- Relax your shoulders away from your ears.

Hold the Pose
- Stay in the pose for five breaths, maintaining steady and deep breathing.

Release the Pose
- Straighten your legs to come out of the squat.
- You can transition directly into a Forward Fold if desired.
- Repeat the pose three times, with other poses in between if practicing at home.

Key Points
- Work towards keeping your feet parallel over time.
- For stability, press your thighs into your upper arms and your upper arms into your thighs.
- Keep your spine straight and chest lifted to avoid rounding the back.

One of the best stretches for those who sit for long periods of time is the spinal figure four, which focuses on the glutes and hips. This stretch helps alleviate stiffness and discomfort in the hips, lower back, and legs and can potentially relieve sciatic pain. By opening the hip joints and muscles, particularly the piriformis, Supine Figure Four promotes better balance and function in the body. Incorporating this stretch into your routine not only enhances physical flexibility but also supports mental health by reducing stress and tension.

Starting Position
- Get into a prone position by bending at the knees and placing your flat feet on the floor.
- Keep your pelvis in a neutral position.

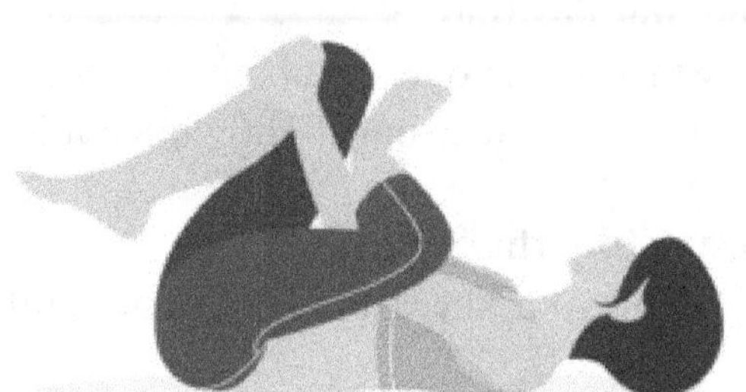

Position the Right Leg
- Lift and open the inner thigh of your right leg.
- Place your right ankle just above your left knee.
- You can stabilize your knee by flexing your right foot, which engages the muscles of your lower thigh.

Lift the Left Leg
- Place both hands behind your left thigh or on your left knee.
- Lift your left leg off the floor, creating a stretch in your right hip and glute muscles.

Deepen the Stretch
- To deepen the stretch, gently press your right knee away from your torso with your right hand.
- Alternatively, place both hands on the back of your left thigh and pull your left leg toward your chest.

Hold the Pose
- Breathe deeply and evenly, holding the stretch for 30 seconds to two minutes.

Release the Pose
- Gently release your hands and return your left foot to the floor.
- Lower your right leg back to the starting position.

Switch Sides
- Repeat the stretch on the opposite side by lifting and positioning your left leg over your right knee.

Key Points
- Flex your foot to support the knee and enhance the stretch.
- Maintain deep, even breaths to help relax and deepen the stretch.
- Ensure your pelvis remains in a neutral position to avoid strain on the lower back.

Hero Pose (Virasana) is a classic seated yoga posture that provides a deep stretch to the thighs, knees, and ankles while promoting a sense of calm and grounding. This pose is often used in meditation and pranayama practice due to its stable and comfortable sitting position. It helps improve posture, relieves fatigue in the legs, and can be beneficial for those with digestive issues. Practicing Hero Pose regularly can also enhance flexibility in the lower body and prepare you for more advanced seated poses.

Starting Position
- Kneel on the floor: Start by kneeling on your yoga mat with your knees together and your thighs perpendicular to the floor.
- Sit back on your heels: Keep your inner thighs close together, and sit back on your heels. Ensure that the tops of your feet are flat on the floor and your toes are pointing straight back.

Adjust Your Feet and Knees
- Separate your feet: Move your feet slightly wider than your hips, ensuring that your toes are still pointing back and the tops of your feet are pressing into the mat.
- Sit between your feet: Slowly lower your buttocks to the floor, sitting between your feet. If this is uncomfortable or if your buttocks do not reach the floor, place a block or blanket under your sit bones for support.

Find Your Alignment
- Lengthen your spine: Sit up tall, lengthening your spine. Ensure your shoulders are directly over your hips and your head is aligned with your spine.
- Rest your hands: Place your hands on your thighs, palms facing down. Relax your shoulders away from your ears and keep your chest open.

Hold the Pose
- Engage your core: Engage your core muscles to support your lower back and maintain a straight posture.
- Breathe deeply: Take slow, deep breaths, inhaling and exhaling through your nose. Hold the pose for 1-5 minutes, gradually increasing the duration as you become more comfortable.

Key Points
- Ensure your knees are together and your feet are separated just enough to allow your sit bones to rest on the floor or a prop.
- Engage your core and lengthen your spine to avoid slouching or rounding your back.
- If you feel discomfort in your knees or ankles, use a block or blanket under your sit bones for support.

Variations:

Starting Position
- Begin in Hero Pose: Start by sitting in Hero Pose with your buttocks on the floor or a prop.

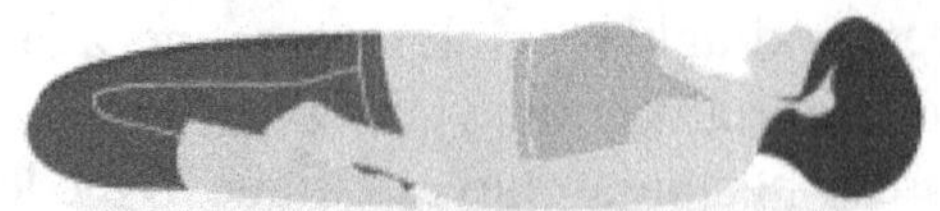

Lean Back
- Support your back: Place your hands on the floor behind you, fingers pointing towards your feet.
- Lower onto your elbows: Slowly lean back, coming down onto your elbows. Pause here if you feel a deep stretch.

Fully Recline
- Lower your back: If comfortable, continue lowering your back to the floor. You can use a bolster or pillows under your back and head for support.
- Adjust your arms: Rest your arms alongside your body, palms facing up.

Hold the Pose
- Breathe deeply: Take slow, deep breaths, relaxing into the pose. Hold for 1-5 minutes.

Extended Reclining Hero Pose

Starting Position
- Begin in Reclining Hero Pose: Start by lying on your back in Reclining Hero Pose with your knees bent and feet beside your hips.

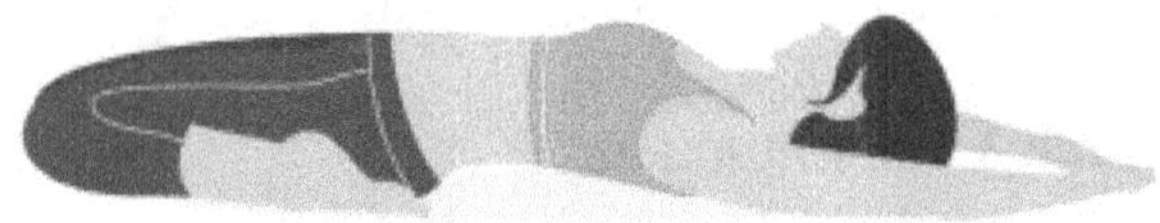

Extend Your Arms and Legs
- Stretch your arms: Extend your arms overhead, reaching towards the wall behind you. Keep your palms facing up.
- Straighten your legs: If comfortable, straighten your legs out in front of you, one at a time. Keep your feet flexed and your legs active.

Find Your Alignment
- Lengthen your spine: Ensure your back is fully supported and your spine is lengthened.
- Adjust your arms: Keep your arms extended, with your shoulders relaxed and away from your ears.

Hold the Pose
- Breathe deeply: Take deep breaths, feeling the stretch along your entire body. Hold for 1-5 minutes.

Lizard Pose (Utthan Pristhasana) is a deep, hip-opening yoga pose that stretches the hamstrings, hip flexors, and quadriceps. In Sanskrit, "Utthan" means to stretch out, "Pristha" means the page of a book, and "Asana" means pose. This pose can be quite intense for the hips, especially if you are less flexible, but modified versions can make it accessible to all levels. Lizard Pose offers numerous benefits, including improving flexibility and strength in the hips and hamstrings, alleviating lower back pain, reducing stress, and enhancing focus and creativity. It is particularly recommended for athletes and those looking to improve their reproductive health by activating the pelvis and lower abdomen.

Starting Position

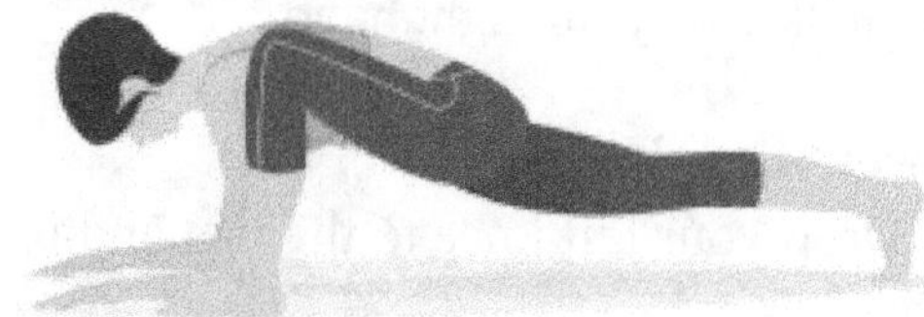

- Begin in Downward-Facing Dog (Adho Mukha Svanasana). Inhale deeply.

Step Forward

- Exhale as you step your right foot to the outside of your right hand. Ensure your foot reaches the front of your mat with your toes in line with your fingers. Your right knee should be bent at a 90-degree angle and stacked above the ankle, with toes pointing out about 45 degrees.

Lower to Forearms

- Inhale as you bring your elbows to the floor with your forearms flat on the mat. Spread your palms out on the floor. Use a block under the forearms if necessary.

Keep Head Neutral

- Keep your head in a neutral, relaxed position.

Engage Back Leg

- Exhale and press into your left heel to keep your left leg active. This helps ensure your hips don't sag toward the floor.

Hold the Pose

- Stay in this position for 5 deep, full breaths.

Release the Pose

- To release, exhale deeply and straighten your arms so your wrists are under your shoulders. Inhale and step back to Downward Dog.

Repeat on the Other Side

- Stay in Downward Dog for several breaths, then repeat the steps starting with your left leg forward to ensure the pose is performed equally on both sides.

Key Points

- Ensure your front knee is stacked above your ankle and your back leg is active to prevent hips from sagging.
- Use a block under your forearms if needed to maintain proper alignment and avoid straining.
- Maintain deep, full breaths throughout the pose to enhance the stretch and relaxation.

Variation:

Modified Lizard Pose with Knee Down

Starting Position
- Begin in Downward-Facing Dog.

Step Forward
- Exhale as you step your right foot to the outside of your right hand.

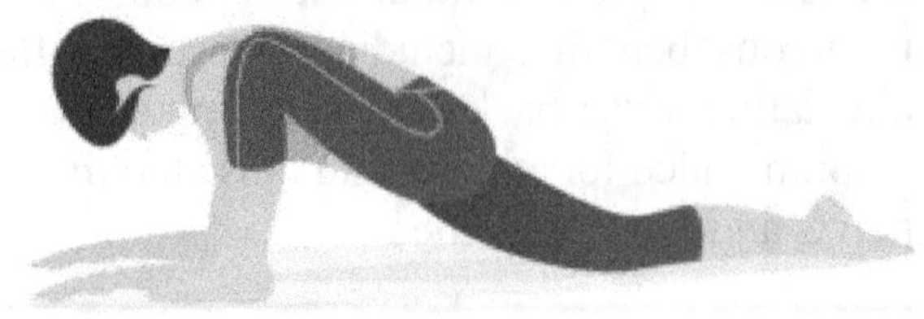

Lower Back Knee
- Drop your left knee to the mat and untuck your toes.

Forearm Support
- Bring your elbows to the floor or onto blocks for support.

Engage Hips
- Press your hips gently forward to deepen the stretch.

Hold the Pose
- Stay for 5 deep, full breaths.

Release the Pose
- To release, straighten your arms, lift your back knee, and step back to Downward Dog.

Repeat
- Repeat on the other side.

Monkey Pose (Hanumanasana) is a deep and intense hip opener that resembles a full split. Named after the Hindu deity Hanuman, who is said to have made a giant leap from India to Sri Lanka, this pose symbolizes a leap of faith, courage, and devotion. Practicing Hanumanasana can help improve flexibility in the hamstrings, hip flexors, and groin while also enhancing mental focus and perseverance. It is an advanced posture that requires preparation and patience to achieve safely.

Starting Position

- Begin in a low lunge: Start in a low lunge position with your right foot forward and your left knee on the ground. Ensure your right knee is directly above your right ankle.
- Hands-on the floor: Place your hands on the floor on either side of your right foot for support.

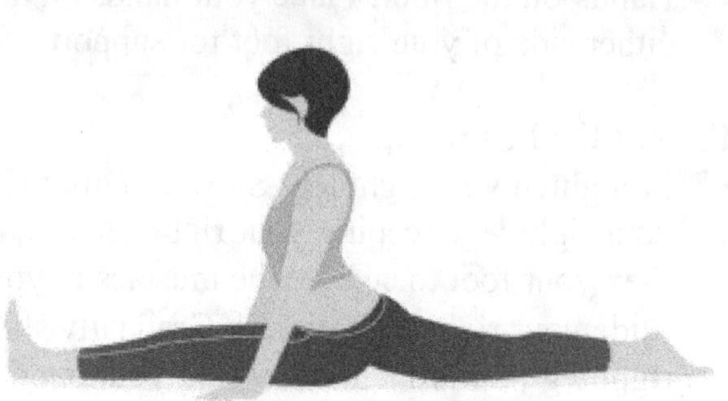

Extend the Front Leg

- Straighten your right leg: Slowly begin to straighten your right leg, keeping your right heel on the floor. Flex your foot to engage the muscles in your leg.
- Slide your right leg forward: Gradually slide your right leg forward while keeping your hands on the floor for support.

Extend the Back Leg

- Slide your left leg back: As you slide your right leg forward, start to slide your left leg back, allowing your hips to lower toward the floor.
- Point your left toes: Keep your left foot pointed and your left leg straight.

Find Your Balance

- Square your hips: Ensure your hips are squared to the front, not tilting to one side.
- Hands on the floor or props: Keep your hands on the floor or use blocks for support as you lower your hips closer to the floor.

Full Expression

- Arms overhead: If you are comfortable and stable, you can raise your arms overhead, bringing your palms together in a prayer position.
- Hold the pose: Breathe deeply and hold the pose for 5-10 breaths, gradually increasing the duration as you become more comfortable.

Key Points

- Ensure your hips are squared to the front to maintain proper alignment and avoid strain.
- Take your time to ease into the pose, using props like blocks to support your hands and maintain balance.
- Engage the muscles in your legs and core to support the deep stretch and prevent injury.

Variation:

Starting Position

- Begin in a low lunge: Start in a low lunge position with your right foot forward and your left knee on the ground. Ensure your right knee is directly above your right ankle.
- Hands-on the floor: Place your hands on the floor on either side of your right foot for support.

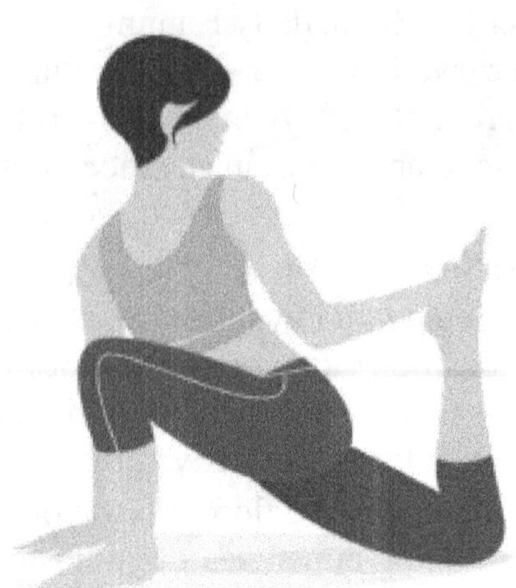

Extend the Front Leg

- Straighten your right leg: Slowly begin to straighten your right leg, keeping your right heel on the floor. Flex your foot to engage the muscles in your leg.
- Slide your right leg forward: Gradually slide your right leg forward while keeping your hands on the floor for support.

Extend the Back Leg

- Slide your left leg back: As you slide your right leg forward, start to slide your left leg back, allowing your hips to lower toward the floor.
- Point your left toes: Keep your left foot pointed and your left leg straight.

Twist the Torso

- Place left hand on the floor: Bring your left hand to the floor for support.
- Reach right arm up Inhale and twist your torso to the right, reaching your right arm up toward the ceiling.

Find Your Balance

- Square your hips: Ensure your hips are squared to the front as much as possible while maintaining the twist.
- Hold the pose: Breathe deeply and hold the pose for 5-10 breaths, gradually increasing the duration as you become more comfortable.

Mermaid Pose is a deep hip opener and backbend that not only stretches the hip flexors, quadriceps, and psoas but also enhances the flexibility of the spine and shoulders. This advanced variation of Pigeon Pose (Eka Pada Rajakapotasana) requires strength, balance, and flexibility. It is an excellent pose for improving posture, increasing the range of motion, and stimulating the nervous system. Practicing Mermaid Pose can also help in releasing deep-seated tension and emotions, providing a sense of liberation and openness.

Starting Position

- Begin in Pigeon Pose: Start in Downward-Facing Dog (Adho Mukha Svanasana). Bring your right knee towards your right wrist, placing your right foot near your left groin. Extend your left leg back, keeping your hips square to the mat.

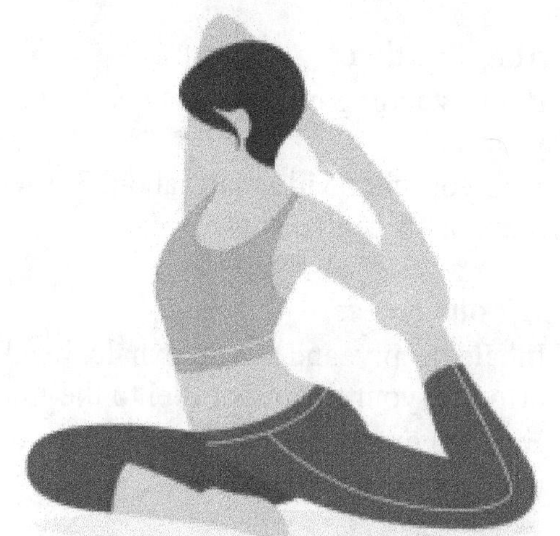

Bend the Back Knee

- Bend the Left Knee: Bend your left knee, bringing your left foot towards your left buttock.

Reach Back with the Arm

- Left Arm Back: Reach your left arm back and hold your left foot or ankle.

Lift the Torso

- Lift the Torso and Right Arm: Lift your torso upright and raise your right arm towards the ceiling.

Create the Bind

- Bind with the Elbow: Bend your left elbow, bringing your left foot closer to your torso. Hook your left foot in the crook of your left elbow.

Hold the Pose

- Stay and Breathe: Hold the pose for 5-10 deep breaths, lengthening the spine and opening the chest with each inhale.

Key Points

- Ensure your hips are square to the mat to maximize the stretch and prevent injury.
- Focus on lifting and opening the chest to deepen the backbend.
- Use your breath to maintain stability and deepen the stretch with each exhalation.

Goddess Pose, or Utkata Konasana, is a powerful standing pose that combines strength, flexibility, and balance. It is often referred to as the "fierce angle pose" due to its intense nature and the strength required to hold the position. This pose is particularly beneficial for opening the hips, strengthening the legs, and toning the core. It also helps improve balance and concentration. Practicing Goddess Pose can instill a sense of empowerment and confidence, making it a favorite in many yoga sequences.

Starting Position
- Begin standing in Tadasana (Mountain Pose) at the center of your mat.
- Step your feet wide apart, about 3-4 feet, turning your toes out to a 45-degree angle.

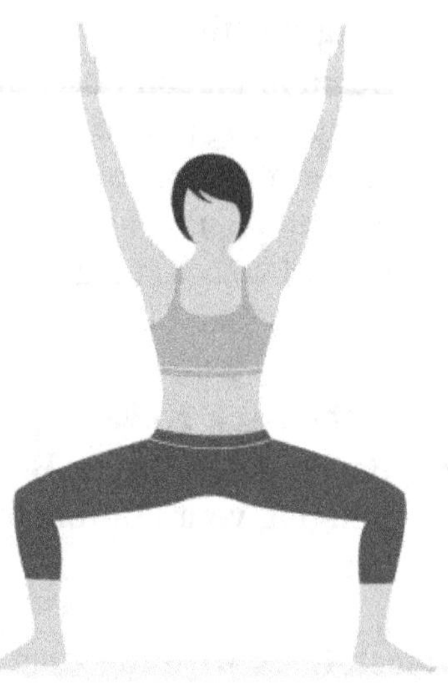

Bend Your Knees
- Inhale deeply, and as you exhale, bend your knees deeply, bringing your thighs parallel to the floor.
- Ensure your knees are aligned over your ankles and they do not extend beyond your toes.

Position Your Arms
- Extend your arms out to the sides at shoulder height, with your palms facing down.
- Bend your elbows to 90 degrees, with your fingertips pointing toward the ceiling in a goalpost position.

Engage and Hold
- Engage your core and draw your tailbone slightly down to avoid overarching your lower back.
- Press your knees out towards your little toes and sink deeper into the pose.
- Hold the pose for 5-10 breaths, maintaining a steady and deep breathing rhythm.

Return to Standing
- Inhale and straighten your legs, bringing your arms back down to your sides.
- Step your feet back together, returning to Tadasana.

Key Points
- Ensure your knees are aligned directly over your ankles and do not extend beyond your toes to protect your joints.
- Engage your core muscles to support your lower back and maintain proper posture.
- Maintain a steady and deep breathing rhythm to help hold the pose and stay focused.

Variation:

Starting in Goddess Pose

- Begin in Goddess Pose with your feet wide apart, knees bent, and arms in the goalpost position.

Twist Your Torso

- Inhale deeply, and as you exhale, twist your torso to the right.
- Bring your left elbow towards your right knee, keeping your right arm extended and fingertips pointing toward the ceiling.
- Ensure your knees stay aligned over your ankles and your lower body remains stable.

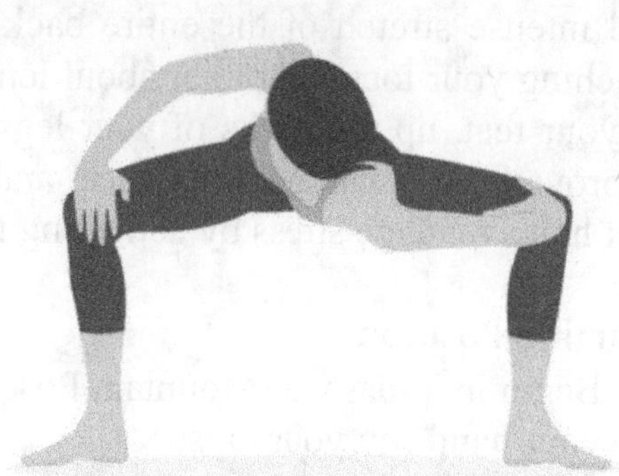

Hold the Twist

- Hold the twisted position for 3-5 breaths, deepening the twist with each exhale.
- Keep your core engaged and your spine long.

Return to Center

- Inhale and return to the center, straightening your torso back to the starting position in Goddess Pose.

Repeat on the Other Side

- Exhale and twist your torso to the left, bringing your right elbow towards your left knee.
- Hold for 3-5 breaths, then return to the center.

Return to Standing

- Inhale, straighten your legs and bring your arms back down to your sides.
- Step your feet back together, returning to Tadasana.

Standing Forward Bend (Uttanasana)

Standing Forward Bend, or Uttanasana, is a foundational yoga pose that emphasizes a deliberate and intense stretch of the entire back body. Contrary to popular belief, this pose is not about touching your toes but rather about lengthening the muscles and connective tissue from the soles of your feet, up the backs of your legs, through your spine, and over your head. Uttanasana can improve body awareness, balance, and flexibility. It also serves as a calming and relaxing pose that helps manage stress by activating the parasympathetic nervous system.

Starting Position
- Begin in Tadasana (Mountain Pose) at the front of your mat with your hands on your hips.

Hinge from the Hips
- In this position, you should bend at the knees and fold your torso over your legs, bending at the hips rather than the lower back.

Place Your Hands
- Let your hands land next to your feet or on the ground in front of you.

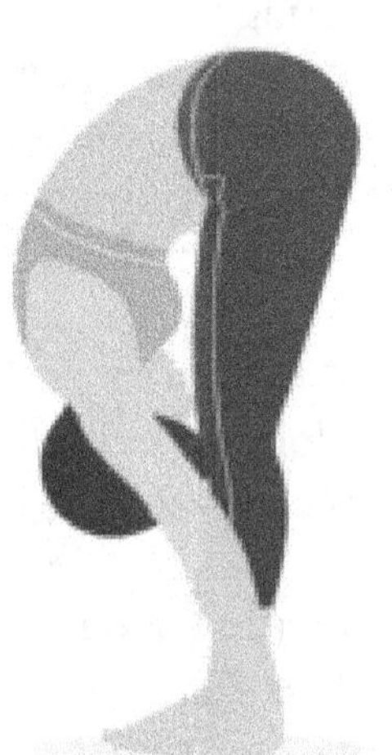

Lengthen Your Spine
- To open up your back, take a deep breath in and widen your chest to stretch your spine.

Straighten Your Legs
- Relax and press both legs forward without hyperextending. Softly spiral your upper and inner thighs back after lifting the kneecaps.

Extend Your Torso
- Exhale and lower your torso without rounding your back. Stretch your neck, extending your head toward the ground and drawing your shoulders down to your hips.

Hold and Breathe
- Hold the posture for a few breaths, inhaling deeply and steadily.

Release the Pose
- Exit the pose by bringing your body back up to Tadasana with a little bend in the knees, hands on hips, and a slow inhalation.

Key Points
- Ensure the movement originates from the hips, not the lower back.
- Keep your spine long and avoid rounding your back.
- Gently press your legs straight and lift your kneecaps to engage your thighs.

Standing Forward Bend (Uttanasana) with Blocks

Start in Tadasana
- Stand at the front of your mat in Mountain Pose.

Place Blocks
- Place yoga blocks in front of your feet at the desired height.

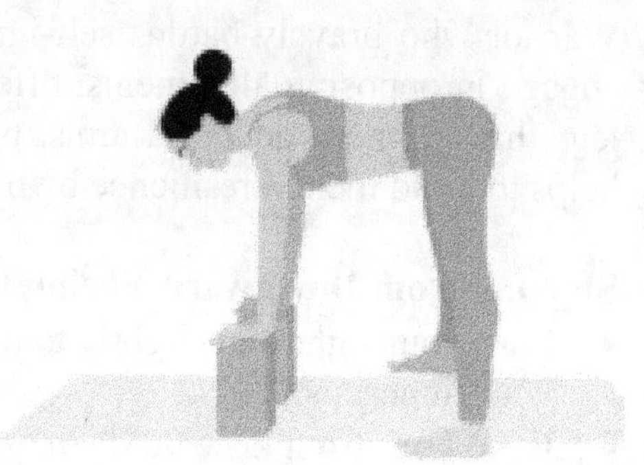

Hinge from the Hips
- Bend your knees slightly and fold your torso over your legs, hanging from the hips.

Hands-on Blocks
- Place your hands on the blocks, keeping your elbows bent as needed.

Press Down
- Focus on pressing down through the balls of your feet to maintain balance.

Lengthen Your Spine
- Inhale and extend your chest to lengthen your spine, then exhale and fold deeper.

Hold and Breathe
- Stay in the pose for several breaths, maintaining deep and steady breathing.

Warrior I, or Virabhadrasana I, is a powerful and dynamic yoga pose that challenges both the body and mind. Named after the mythical Warrior Virabhadra, this pose symbolizes the inner spiritual Warrior who bravely battles self-ignorance, the root of all suffering. Warrior I requires you to engage in opposing alignments, offering a full-body experience. It strengthens and stretches the legs, hips, upper body, and arms, promoting balance, focus, and determination. This pose also helps to build mental resilience by pushing past perceived limitations.

Starting from Downward-Facing Dog (Adho Mukha Svanasana)

- Shift your right foot slightly to the right until your toes touch your fingertips.
- Bend your front knee 90 degrees, thigh parallel to the floor, knee over ankle.

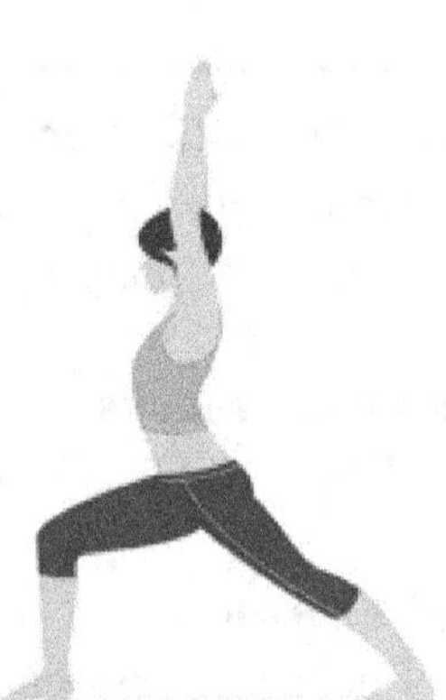

Position Your Back Foot

- Make a 45-degree curve with your foot by turning your left heel to the floor.
- Place your feet slightly wider or align your left and right heels for stability.
- Press your left thighbone back, keeping your left knee straight.

Raise Your Torso and Arms

- Elevate your torso and lift your arms shoulder-distance apart with palms facing each other.
- Open your shoulder blades away from your spine and toward your outer armpits.
- Bend at the elbows and pull in your triceps to your midline. It is acceptable to stare up at your thumbs while bringing your hands together.

Engage Your Core and Legs

- As you let your tailbone fall toward the floor, maintain forcing your left femur back.
- Separate your right thigh from your lower tummy by drawing it back and up.

Hold the Pose

- Hold for 5–10 breaths, maintaining deep and steady breathing.

Release the Pose

- Exhale, drop your hands, return to Downward-Facing Dog, and repeat on the opposite side.

Key Points

- Put the front knee directly over the ankle and the back foot at 45 degrees.
- Draw the lower belly back and up to support the spine.
- Keep shoulder blades open and arms reaching up while maintaining space between the shoulders and ears.

Variation:

Starting Position
- Sit on a chair: Sit sideways on a chair with the right side of your body facing the back of the chair. Ensure your feet are flat on the floor and your knees are bent at 90 degrees.

Position the Legs
- Extend left leg: Slide your left leg back behind you, straightening it fully. Your left foot should be flat on the floor with the toes pointing slightly inward.
- Bend right knee: Keep your right knee bent at 90 degrees, with your right foot flat on the floor and pointing forward.

Position the Arms
- Raise your arms: Extend your arms overhead, parallel to each other, with your palms facing inward.

Align the Torso
- Square your hips: Ensure your hips are squared to the front of the chair and your torso is upright.
- Lift your chest: Slightly lift your chest and gaze forward or up at your hands if comfortable.

Hold the Pose
- Breathe deeply: Stay in this position for 5-10 breaths, maintaining the alignment of your legs, hips, and arms.

Switch Sides
- Repeat on the other side: Turn around to sit on the other side of the chair and repeat the steps with your left leg forward.

Warrior II, or Virabhadrasana II, is a powerful standing pose that enhances strength, stamina, and focus. This posture represents bravery and resolve, and it is named after the ferocious Hindu hero Virabhadra. In Warrior II, the front knee bends deeply, the arms extend powerfully out from the shoulders, and the gaze is directed calmly over the front hand. The legs, hips, core, and shoulders all get a workout in with this position, which also helps with balance and endurance. It's a vital pose for building physical resilience and mental fortitude, helping practitioners tap into their inner strength and focus.

Face the Long Side of Your Mat
- Stand with your feet wide apart, about double hip-width distance.
- With palms down, extend your arms straight out from your shoulders, parallel to the floor.

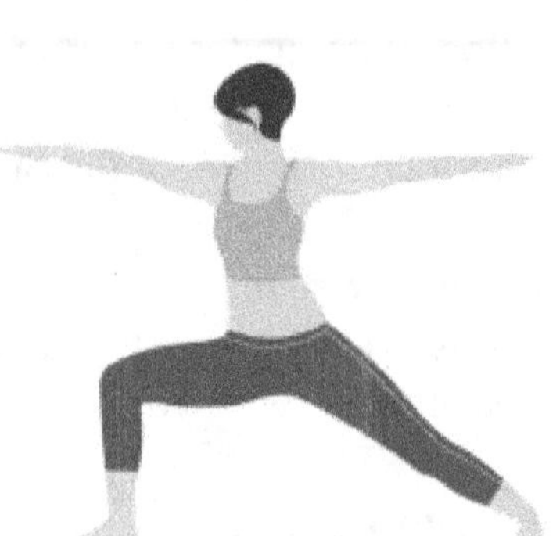

Align Your Feet
- Turn your right foot to face the front of the mat.
- Angle your left toes slightly inward toward the upper left corner of the mat.

Bend Your Front Knee
- Bend your right knee, stacking it over your right ankle.
- Keep your thigh parallel to the floor and knee 90 degrees.

Engage Your Legs
- Distribute weight evenly between legs.
- Press through your back foot's outer edge.

Align Your Torso and Arms
- Hold your head over your pelvis and shoulders over your hips.
- Both arms should extend powerfully to the mat's front and back.

Find Your Gaze
- Turn your head to look past your right fingertips, maintaining a calm and steady gaze.

Hold the Pose
- Stay in the pose for 5-10 breaths, keeping your breathing deep and steady.

Release the Pose
- Exhale as you press down through your feet.
- Inhale and straighten your legs, returning your feet to parallel facing the long side of the mat.

Switch Sides
- Repeat the pose on the other side.

Key Points

- Ensure your front knee is stacked over your ankle and your back foot is angled slightly inward.
- Distribute weight evenly and engage your core to support the pose.
- Maintain a steady gaze over your front hand to help with balance and focus.

Variation:

Warrior II with a Chair

Starting Position

- Sit on a chair: Sit sideways on a chair with the right side of your body facing the back of the chair. Ensure your feet are flat on the floor and your knees are bent at 90 degrees.

Position the Legs

- Extend left leg: Slide your left leg back behind you, straightening it fully. Your left foot should
- be flat on the floor with the toes pointing slightly inward.
- Bend right knee: Keep your right knee bent at 90 degrees, with your right foot flat on the floor and pointing forward.

Position the Arms

- Raise your arms: Extend your arms straight out from your shoulders, parallel to the floor, with your palms facing down.

Align the Torso

- Square your hips: Ensure your hips are squared to the side of the chair and your torso is upright.
- Gaze forward: Turn your head to look over your right fingertips.

Hold the Pose

- Breathe deeply: Stay in this position for 5-10 breaths, maintaining the alignment of your legs, hips, and arms.

Switch Sides

- Repeat on the other side: Turn around to sit on the other side of the chair and repeat the steps with your left leg forward.

Warrior III, or Virabhadrasana III, is a powerful standing balance pose that requires concentration, stamina, and a thoughtful calibration between push and pull. Named after the warrior Virabhadra from Hindu mythology, this pose challenges you to stay grounded on one leg while extending the other leg and your arms horizontally, creating a sense of expansion and contraction simultaneously. This dynamic balance pose strengthens your core and legs and improves overall stability and coordination. Warrior III is a testament to the power and resilience of a true warrior, encouraging mental focus and physical strength.

Begin in Warrior I
- Start with your right foot forward in Warrior I (Virabhadrasana I).

Engage and Root
- Root down firmly with your right heel, lifting your lower belly and drawing the abdominals in and up.
- Release your tailbone down.

Align and Energize
- Hold your right outer hip in your midline and straighten your left leg.
- In order to bring your side body to a longer length, energize your arms.

Prepare for the Transition
- Roll your left outer hip forward by turning your left inner thigh to the ceiling.
- Pivot onto your back toes, bringing your back leg into a neutral position.

Tilt and Reach
- Inhale to lengthen your spine.
- Exhale, tilt your torso forward and extend your arms.

Lift and Balance
- Lift your left leg to floor level and shift your weight into your front foot.
- Your upper arms should frame your ears and your head, torso, pelvis, and elevated leg should be straight.

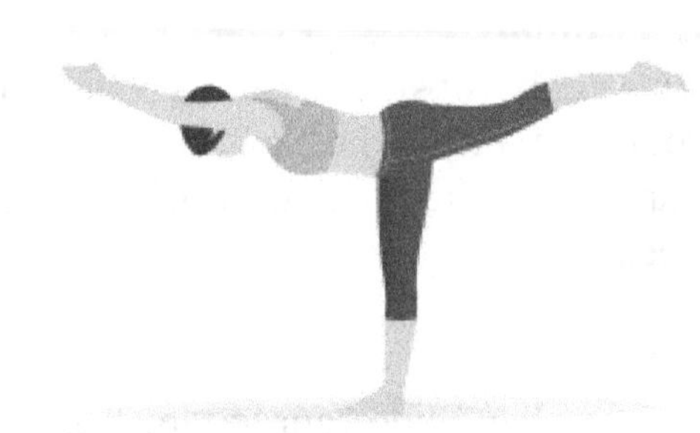

Maintain Alignment
- Continue turning your left inner thigh to the ceiling to keep your leg neutral and your pelvis level.
- Engage your right outer hip for stability.

Extend and Hold
- Stretch your arms, crown, and sternum forward while pushing back with your left heel.
- Tone your lower belly and tailbone toward your left heel for lower back support.

Breathe and Release
- Hold the pose for 5–10 breaths, maintaining deep and steady breathing.
- Bend your right knee and step back to Warrior I with your left foot.
- Repeat on the other side.

Key Points
- Ensure your body forms a straight line from your fingertips to your lifted heel.
- Keep your lower belly toned to support your lower back and maintain balance.
- Maintain a steady gaze to help with balance and focus.

Variation:

Starting Position
- Stand facing the wall: Position yourself about a foot away from a wall, standing in Tadasana (Mountain Pose) with your feet hip-width apart.

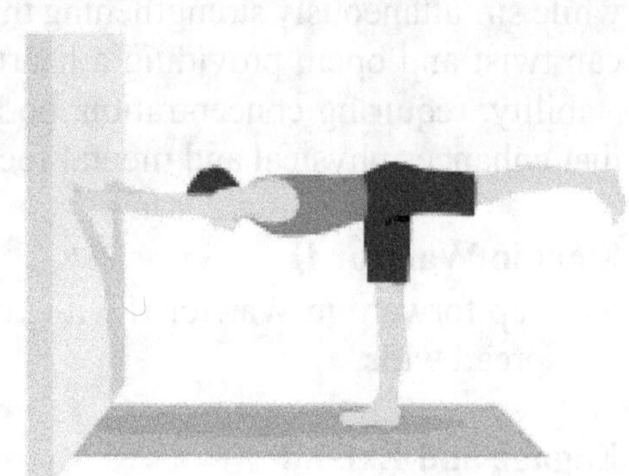

Extend the Arms
- Reach forward: Extend your arms forward and place your palms flat against the wall at shoulder height, keeping your arms straight.

Position the Legs
- Step back with one leg: Step your left foot back, keeping your right foot firmly planted on the ground.
- Shift weight: Begin to shift your weight onto your right foot, preparing to lift your left leg.

Lift the Leg
- Raise the left leg: As you hinge forward from your hips, lift your left leg behind you, keeping it straight and in line with your torso. Your body should form a straight line from your fingertips to your left heel.

Align the Torso
- Square your hips: Ensure your hips are squared to the ground. Engage your core to maintain balance and stability.
- Lengthen the spine: Keep your back straight, extending through the crown of your head and reaching out through your lifted heel.

Adjust the Position
- Fine-tune alignment: Use the wall for balance, adjusting your position as needed to maintain a straight line from your hands to your lifted foot.
- Flex the lifted foot: Flex your left foot, keeping it active and engaged.

Hold the Pose
- Breathe deeply: Stay in this position for 5-10 breaths, focusing on maintaining your balance and alignment.

Return to Starting Position
- Lower the leg: Slowly lower your left leg back to the ground, returning to an upright position.
- Step forward: Step your left foot forward to meet your right foot, returning to Tadasana.

Switch Sides
- Repeat on the other side: Turn around and repeat the steps with your right leg lifted.

Utthita Trikonasana, or Triangle Pose, is an essential yoga pose that is practiced in virtually all schools of yoga. This pose offers a powerful stretch for the hamstrings, groin, hips, and shoulders while simultaneously strengthening the legs. By grounding the feet and engaging the legs, the chest can twist and open, providing a heart-opening expansion. Triangle Pose challenges balance and stability, requiring concentration, body awareness, and a steady breath, making it a holistic pose that enhances physical and mental focus.

Start in Warrior II
- Step forward in Warrior II with your right foot and arms spread wide.

Engage and Extend
- Pull your right femur into its socket with your right thigh.
- Cross your right leg over your left and bring your right hand up to your face.

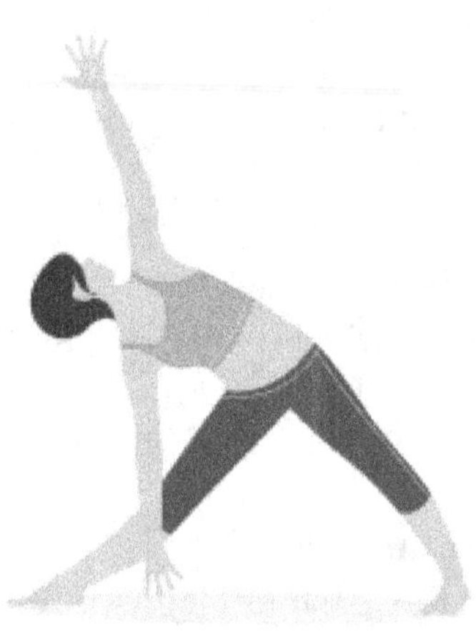

Lower and Align
- Lower your right hand down onto your shin, ankle, or the floor inside or outside your right foot, depending on your flexibility and comfort.
- Place your left shoulder on top of your right, open your chest, and stretch your left fingertips to the ceiling while retaining your left shoulder in its socket.

Adjust Your Gaze
- Look up at your left fingertips. If this hurts your neck, keep your head neutral.

Maintain Alignment
- Keep drawing your right thigh muscles up, deepening your right hip crease. A microbead can soften your right knee to prevent hyperextension.

Hold the Pose
- Stay in this position for at least 5 breaths, maintaining deep and steady breathing.

Release and Repeat
- Inhale and stand up to exit the posture. Repeat the position with your left leg forward after exhaling.

Key Points
- Ensure your body forms various-sized triangles with your legs and arms.
- Engage your thigh muscles and keep your shoulders aligned.
- Maintain a steady breath to help focus and balance.

Variation:

Starting Position

- Stand in Tadasana: Begin in Mountain Pose with your feet together and arms at your sides.
- Separate your legs: Step your feet about 3-4 feet apart, aligning your heels.

Position Your Feet

- Turn the right foot out: Turn your right foot to face the short edge of the mat at a 90-degree angle.
- Turn the left foot slightly in Angle your left foot slightly toward the right foot at about 45 degrees.

Align Your Body

- Lift through the spine: Inhale and stretch your arms out to the sides, parallel to the floor, palms facing down.
- Engage your legs: Firm your thigh muscles and ground both feet into the mat.

Hinge at the Hips

- Reach forward: Extend your right arm forward, reaching as far as you can while keeping your left hip back.
- Lower your right hand: Place your right hand on a brick positioned behind your right shin, on the inside or outside of your right foot. Adjust the height of the brick to a comfortable level.

Extend the Left Arm

- Reach up: Extend your left arm straight up towards the ceiling, aligning it with your shoulders.
- Open your chest: Turn your head to look at your left thumb, or keep your head in a neutral position if that is more comfortable.

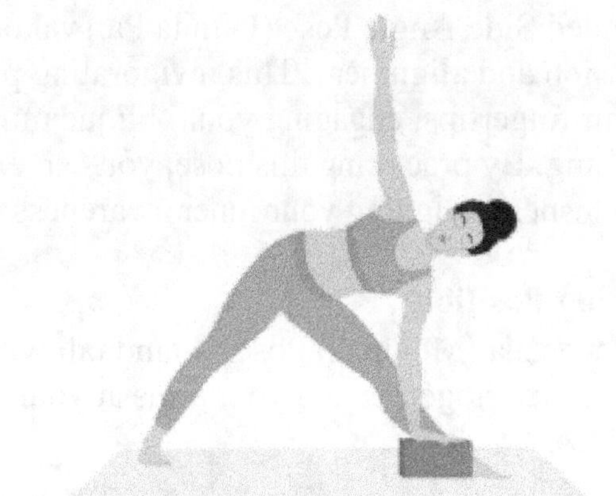

Adjust Your Alignment

- Check your hips: Ensure your hips are open, with the left hip stacked over the right hip.
- Lengthen your spine: Keep your spine long and straight, avoiding any rounding in the back.

Hold the Pose

- Breathe deeply: Stay in this position for 5-10 breaths, focusing on maintaining your balance and alignment.
- Engage the core: Draw your navel in towards your spine to support your lower back.

Return to Starting Position

- Inhale to rise: Press firmly into your feet and lift your torso back up to standing, arms extended out to the sides.
- Lower your arms: Bring your arms back down to your sides.

Switch Sides

- Repeat on the other side: Turn your left foot out and your right foot in, and repeat the steps with your left hand on the brick and right arm extended.

Extended Side Angle Pose (Utthita Parsvakonasana) is a powerful yoga posture that emphasizes extension and alignment. This invigorating pose stretches your entire body, from your outer heel to your fingertips, engaging your oblique muscles and opening your rib cage to encourage deeper breathing. By practicing this pose, you can expand your sense of self and create a feeling of spaciousness, aligning your inner awareness with the universal space around you.

Starting Position

- Tadasana (Mountain Pose): Stand tall with your feet together and your arms at your sides.

Jump to Stance

- Jump Your Legs Apart Jump your legs about 4 feet apart, extending your arms into a T position with palms facing down.

Foot Placement

- Adjust Your Feet: Turn your left foot out 90 degrees and turn your right foot slightly inward.

Bend the Knee

- Bend the Left Knee Bend your left knee towards a 90-degree angle, ensuring your left thigh is parallel to the floor.

Lean and Reach

- Lean to the Left. Lean towards your left knee, hinging at the hips. Place your left arm on the floor or a block inside or outside your left foot.

Arm Extension

- Extend the Right Arm: Reach your right arm over your right ear, palm facing down. Turn your chest towards your raised arm,

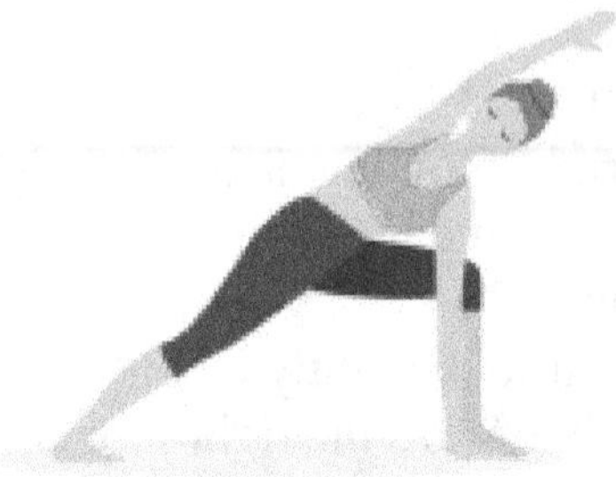

creating a straight line from your right ankle to your right hand.

Head Position

- Turn Your Head Turn your head to look past your right thumb.

Breathe

- Hold the Pose. Stay in this position for 30 to 60 seconds, breathing freely.

Switch Sides

- Come Up and Switch. Inhale as you reach up and straighten your left leg. Switch sides and repeat the pose on the other side.

Key Points

- Ensure your hips and chest are open, maintaining a straight line from your back heel to your fingertips.
- Keep your front knee directly above your ankle, and press firmly through both feet.
- Extend your top arm and torso, creating length and space in your side body.

Variation:

Starting Position
- Stand in Tadasana: Begin in Mountain Pose with your feet together and arms at your sides.
- Separate your legs: Step your feet about 3-4 feet apart, aligning your heels.

Position Your Feet
- Turn the right foot out: Turn your right foot to face the short edge of the mat at a 90-degree angle.
- Turn the left foot slightly in Angle your left foot slightly toward the right foot at about 45 degrees.

Align Your Body
- Lift through the spine: Inhale and stretch your arms out to the sides, parallel to the floor, palms facing down.
- Engage your legs: Firm your thigh muscles and ground both feet into the mat.

Bend the Right Knee
- Bend your front knee: Exhale and bend your right knee until your thigh is parallel to the floor. Your knee should be directly above your ankle, forming a 90-degree angle.

Hinge at the Hips
- Reach forward: Extend your right arm forward, reaching as far as you can while keeping your left hip back.
- Lower your right hand: Place your right hand on a brick positioned on the inside or outside of your right foot. Adjust the height of the brick to a comfortable level.

Extend the Left Arm
- Reach up and over: Stretch your left arm up towards the ceiling, then extend it over your left ear with your palm facing down.

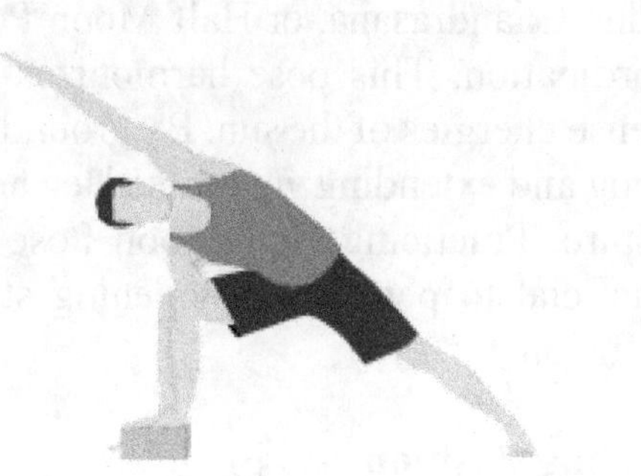

- Open your chest: Turn your chest upward, open the ribcage, and keep your left shoulder back.

Adjust Your Alignment
- Check your hips: Ensure your hips are open, with the left hip stacked over the right hip.
- Lengthen your spine: Keep your spine long and straight, avoiding any rounding in the back.

Hold the Pose
- Breathe deeply: Stay in this position for 5-10 breaths, focusing on maintaining your balance and alignment.
- Engage the core: Draw your navel in towards your spine to support your lower back.

Return to Starting Position
- Inhale to rise: Press firmly into your feet and lift your torso back up to standing, arms extended out to the sides.
- Lower your arms: Bring your arms back down to your sides.

Switch Sides
- Repeat on the other side: Turn your left foot out and your right foot in, and repeat the steps with your left hand on the brick and right arm extended.

Ardha Chandrasana, or Half Moon Pose, is a challenging yoga posture that requires balance and coordination. This pose harmonizes the calming, cooling energies of the moon and the fiery, intense energies of the sun. By grounding through your standing leg and stabilizing your arm while lifting and extending your raised leg and opposite arm, you can achieve a balanced and harmonious posture. Practicing Half Moon Pose on both sides helps correct postural imbalances, and it's beneficial to perform hip-opening stretches beforehand to facilitate torso rotation and ribcage extension.

Starting Position
- Begin in Extended Triangle Pose Start with Utthita Trikonasana (Extended Triangle) with your left foot forward.

Prepare for Balance
- Hand to Hip: Bring your right hand to your hip and turn your head to look at the floor.

Shift Weight
- Shift Forward Bend your front leg and shift your weight into your front foot.

Position Your Hand
- Hand Placement: Reach your front hand a little forward and place it on the mat or a block directly beneath your front shoulder. Press down through your fingers to steady yourself.

Lift the Leg
- Lift and Extend: Lift your back leg until your thigh is parallel to the floor. Slowly turn your chest to face the right, twisting your torso and hips. Reach your top hand to the ceiling.

Adjust Your Gaze
- Gaze Adjustment: Either keep your gaze on the floor or slowly bring it to your top hand. Keep a slight bend in your standing leg to avoid hyperextending your knee.

Variation:

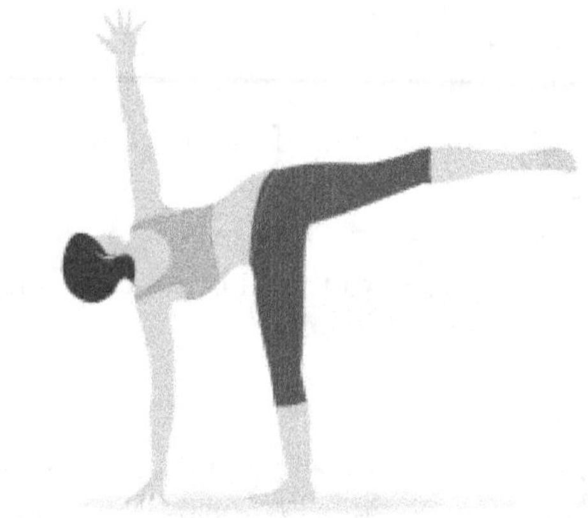

Hold the Pose
- Breathe and Balance: Hold the pose for 5 to 10 breaths, maintaining steady and even breathing.

Exit the Pose
- Return to Triangle Exit the pose the same way you came into it and return to Extended Triangle Pose.

Key Points
- Engage your core and use your fingers to stabilize yourself, keeping your body steady and balanced.
- Ensure your standing leg is slightly bent and your raised leg is parallel to the floor, with your chest open and facing the side.
- Maintain a steady and even breath, using it to help maintain balance and focus.

Use a Wall for Support
- Begin in an Extended Triangle Pose with your back against a wall for added stability.

Shift Forward
- Bend your front leg and shift your weight into your front foot.

Hand Placement
- Place your front hand on a block positioned in front of your foot and against the wall for additional support.

Lift the Leg
- Lift your back leg, keeping your back foot pressing into the wall to maintain balance.

Extend and Reach
- Extend your top hand to the ceiling, keeping your back pressed against the wall.

Hold the Pose
- Hold for 5 to 10 breaths, maintaining steady and even breathing.

Exit the Pose
- Exit the pose the same way you came into it, returning to Extended Triangle Pose.

Wheel Pose, or Urdhva Dhanurasana, is a powerful backbend that opens up the chest, stretches the entire front body, and strengthens the back, arms, and legs. This pose is invigorating and can create a sense of energy and exhilaration. Practicing Wheel Pose can help improve flexibility in the spine and shoulders, as well as build strength in the muscles of the back and arms. It is often included in intermediate to advanced yoga sequences due to its intensity and the strength required.

Starting Position
- Lie on your back: Begin by lying flat on your back with your knees bent and feet flat on the floor, hip-width apart.
- Position your hands: Bend your elbows and place your palms on the floor beside your head, fingers pointing towards your shoulders.

Prepare to Lift
- Engage your legs: Press your feet firmly into the floor and engage your quadriceps.
- Position your arms: Press your hands into the floor, keeping your elbows shoulder-width apart.

Lift the Hips
- Inhale deeply: On an inhale, press into your feet and lift your hips towards the ceiling.
- Lift the chest: Continue pressing into your hands to lift your chest off the floor, coming onto the crown of your head briefly.

Full Expression
- Straighten the arms: Press firmly through your hands to fully extend your arms, lifting your head off the floor and straightening your arms.
- Open the chest: Lift your chest towards the ceiling, drawing your shoulder blades towards your back.
- Engage the legs: Press firmly through your feet, lifting your hips higher and engaging your thighs.

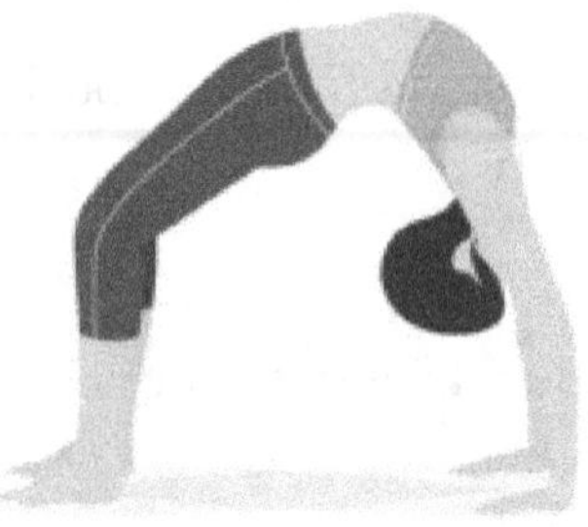

Hold the Pose
- Breathe deeply: Hold the pose for 5-10 breaths, breathing deeply and steadily.
- Stay strong: Keep your legs and arms active to maintain the lift and openness in your chest and spine.

Release the Pose
- Lower down: To come out of the pose, tuck your chin to your chest, bend your elbows, and lower your body gently back to the floor.
- Rest: Hug your knees to your chest and rock gently side to side to release your lower back.

Key Points
- Ensure your feet are hip-width apart and parallel, and your hands are placed firmly with fingers pointing towards your shoulders.
- Actively engage your legs and arms to lift your hips and chest, creating a strong and stable foundation.
- Maintain steady, deep breaths to help sustain the pose and support the backbend.

Variation:

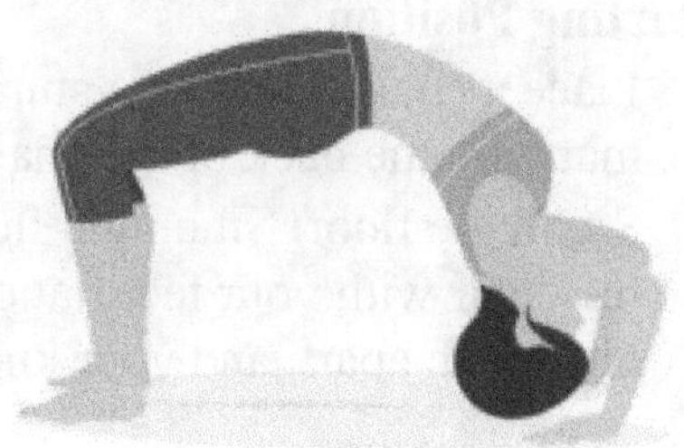

Starting Position

- Stand in Tadasana: Begin by standing tall in Mountain Pose (Tadasana) with your feet hip-width apart and your arms by your sides.
- Engage your core: Activate your core muscles by gently pulling your navel towards your spine.

Position Your Hands

- Place your hands on your lower back: Bring your hands to your lower back with your fingers pointing downwards, providing support as you move into the backbend.
- Draw your elbows together: Squeeze your elbows towards each other to open your chest and lift your heart.

Lift Your Chest

- Inhale and lengthen: Take a deep breath in, lengthening your spine and lifting your chest towards the ceiling.
- Prepare for the backbend: Keep your chin slightly tucked to maintain length in the back of your neck.

Bend Backwards

- Exhale and lean back: As you exhale, gently begin to lean back, using your hands for support. Focus on lifting your chest and keeping your lower back long.
- Maintain your balance: Keep your feet firmly grounded and your thighs engaged to support the backbend.

Deepen the Pose

- Open your chest: Continue to lift your chest and open your heart towards the ceiling. Allow your head to gently fall back if it feels comfortable.
- Engage your legs: Press down through your feet and engage your leg muscles to help stabilize the pose.

Hold the Pose

- Breathe deeply: Stay in the pose for 3-5 deep breaths, allowing your chest to expand with each inhale and soften into the backbend with each exhale.
- Relax your shoulders: Keep your shoulders relaxed and away from your ears.

Release the Pose

- Inhale to come up: On an inhale, engage your core and slowly lift your torso back up to a standing position.
- Return to Tadasana: Bring your arms back to your sides and stand tall in Mountain Pose, taking a few breaths to center yourself.

Starting Position

- Place a chair: Position a sturdy chair on your mat with the back of the chair facing you.
- Sit on the floor: Sit on the floor in front of the chair with your feet flat on the ground, hip-width apart, and your knees bent.

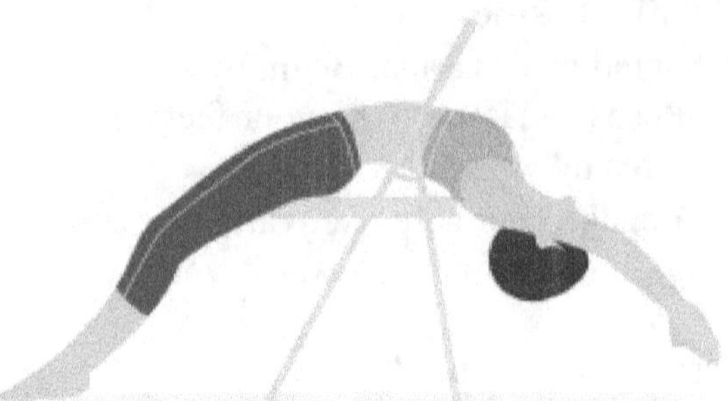

Position Your Hands and Feet

- Place your hands on the chair: Reach your hands back and hold onto the edges of the seat of the chair or the backrest, depending on your flexibility and comfort.
- Feet placement: Ensure your feet are firmly planted on the ground, parallel and hip-width apart.

Lift the Hips

- Inhale deeply: On an inhale, press into your feet and lift your hips towards the ceiling.
- Support with the chair: Use the support of the chair to help lift your chest and create the backbend.

Full Expression

- Extend your arms: Straighten your arms as much as possible while using the chair for support.
- Open the chest: Lift your chest towards the ceiling, drawing your shoulder blades towards your back.
- Engage the legs: Press firmly through your feet, lifting your hips higher and engaging your thighs.

Hold the Pose

- Breathe deeply: Hold the pose for 5-10 breaths, breathing deeply and steadily.
- Stay strong: Keep your legs and arms active to maintain the lift and openness in your chest and spine.

Release the Pose

- Lower down: To come out of the pose, tuck your chin to your chest, bend your elbows, and lower your body gently back to the floor.
- Rest: Hug your knees to your chest and rock gently side to side to release your lower back.

The one-legged Wheel Pose, or Eka Pada Urdhva Dhanurasana, is a powerful and advanced backbend that builds on the foundation of the traditional Wheel Pose. This pose enhances strength, flexibility, and balance while simultaneously engaging the core, back, legs, and shoulders. Incorporating this pose into your practice can help you overcome physical and mental barriers, fostering a deeper connection with your body and improving overall stability and posture.

Starting Position
- Lie on your back with your knees bent and feet flat on the floor, hip-distance apart.
- Place your hands beside your head, fingers pointing toward your shoulders.

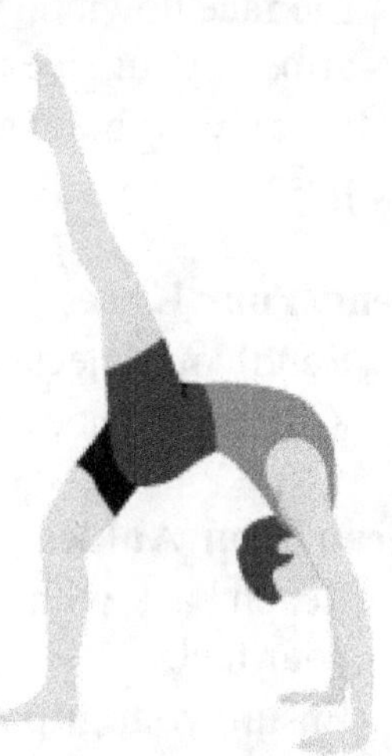

Lift into Wheel Pose
- Inhale deeply, pressing through your hands and feet to lift your hips off the floor.
- Exhale, pressing into your hands and feet to straighten your arms and legs, coming into the full Wheel Pose (Urdhva Dhanurasana).

Prepare for One-Legged Wheel
- Inhale and stabilize your body by pressing firmly through both feet and hands.
- Shift your weight slightly to your left foot.

Lift One Leg
- Exhale as you slowly lift your right foot off the ground, extending your right leg straight up towards the ceiling.
- Keep your hips level and your lifted leg active, pointing your toes or flexing your foot.

Hold the Pose
- Breathe deeply and steadily, maintaining the position for 3-5 breaths.
- Keep your gaze steady, either looking at a fixed point on the ceiling or slightly downwards.

Release the Pose
- Exhale as you slowly lower your right foot back to the ground.
- Inhale to stabilize in the full Wheel Pose.
- Exhale as you gently lower your body back down to the mat, bringing your chin to your chest and releasing your arms and legs.

Repeat on the Other Side
- After resting for a few breaths, repeat the pose on the opposite side, lifting your left leg.

Key Points
- Ensure your supporting foot and both hands are firmly grounded to maintain balance.
- Keep your core muscles active to support your back and maintain alignment.
- Maintain deep, steady breaths to support your balance and focus.

Bow Pose, or Dhanurasana, is a backbend that deeply stretches the chest, shoulders, and thighs while strengthening the back and improving posture. This pose resembles an archer's bow, with your torso and legs representing the body of the bow and your arms the string.

Starting Position
- Lie face down on your mat with your legs extended and your arms at your sides.
- Relax your body and take a few deep breaths to prepare for the pose.

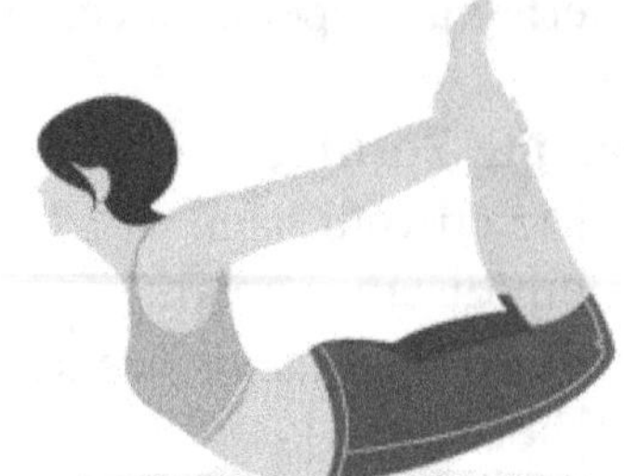

Bend Your Knees
- Bend your knees and bring your heels toward your buttocks.
- Keep your knees hip-width apart to maintain stability and avoid straining your lower back.

Grab Your Ankles
- Reach back with both hands and grab your ankles. If this is difficult, you can grab the tops of your feet.
- Ensure your grip is firm but gentle to avoid any discomfort.

Lift Your Chest and Thighs
- Inhale deeply and simultaneously lift your chest and thighs off the floor.
- Press your ankles into your hands to create a taut bow shape with your body.
- Keep your gaze forward or slightly upward, but avoid compressing your neck.

Hold the Pose
- Hold the pose for 20 to 30 seconds, maintaining steady and deep breathing.
- Focus on lifting your chest higher and bringing your thighs further off the ground with each inhale.

Release
- Exhale and gently lower your chest and thighs back to the floor.
- Release your ankles and rest your arms at your sides.
- Take a few deep breaths to relax and feel the effects of the stretch.

Key Points
- Keep your core engaged to protect your lower back and support the lift.
- Focus on lifting your chest to enhance the stretch in your shoulders and chest.
- Maintain steady and even breathing throughout the pose to help deepen the stretch and maintain balance.

Variations:

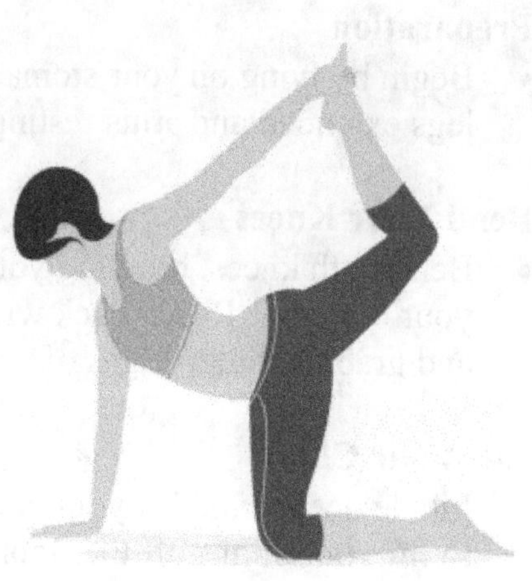

Starting Position
- Lie face down on your mat with your legs extended and your arms at your sides.
- Relax your body and take a few deep breaths.

Bend One Knee
- Bend your right knee and bring your right heel toward your buttock.
- Keep your left leg extended straight on the floor.

Grab Your Ankle
- Reach back with your right hand and grab your right ankle or the top of your foot.
- Keep your grip firm but gentle.

Lift Your Chest and Thigh
- Inhale deeply and lift your chest and right thigh off the floor simultaneously.
- Press your right ankle into your hand to deepen the stretch and lift higher.
- Keep your left leg and arm relaxed on the floor.

Hold the Pose
- Hold the pose for 20 to 30 seconds, maintaining steady and deep breathing.
- Focus on lifting your chest higher with each inhale.

Release and Switch Sides
- Exhale and gently lower your chest and right thigh back to the floor.
- Release your right ankle and rest for a moment.
- Repeat the same steps on the left side, bending your left knee and lifting your left thigh.

Preparation

- Begin by lying on your stomach with your legs extended and arms resting by your sides.

Bend Your Knees

- Bend both knees, bringing your heels toward your buttocks. Reach back with both hands and grab the outer edges of your ankles.

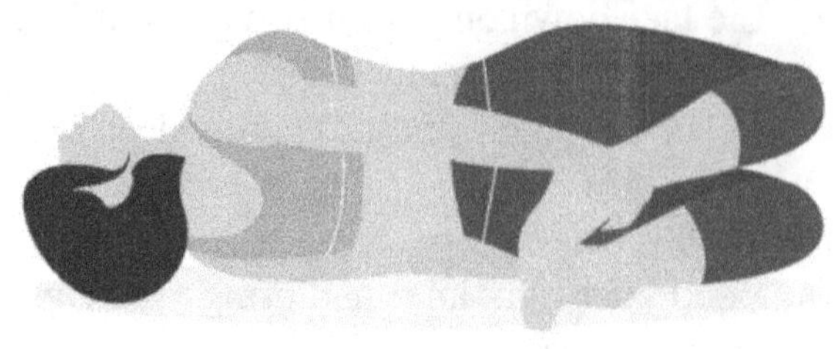

Lift Your Chest

- Inhale deeply and lift your chest off the floor. Simultaneously, pull your ankles up and back to lift your thighs off the floor. This will bring your body into the traditional Bow Pose.

Roll to the Side

- As you exhale, gently roll onto your right side. Use the leverage of your arms and legs to control the movement.

Adjust Your Position

- Keep pulling your ankles back to lift your thighs higher and open your chest more. Your left shoulder should be stacked above your right shoulder and your left hip above your right hip.

Hold the Pose

- Stay in this position for 5-10 breaths. Focus on keeping your balance and maintaining a deep, steady breath.

Return to Center

- To come out of the pose, inhale and gently roll back onto your stomach, returning to the traditional Bow Pose.

Switch Sides

- Exhale and roll onto your left side, following the same steps to ensure both sides are balanced.

Release the Pose

- After holding the pose on the left side for 5-10 breaths, inhale and return to the center. Gently release your grip on your ankles and lower your legs and chest to the floor.

Rest

- Rest your head on your arms and take a few deep breaths to relax and observe the effects of the pose.

Corpse Pose (Savasana)

Corpse Pose (Savasana) is a crucial part of any yoga session, typically practiced at the end to allow the body and mind to absorb the benefits of the asanas. While it appears simple, lying down and relaxing with awareness can be quite challenging. Savasana helps you process the physical and mental effects of your practice, promoting deep relaxation and stress relief. Practicing Savasana regularly can improve your overall sense of well-being and enhance the quality of your sleep.

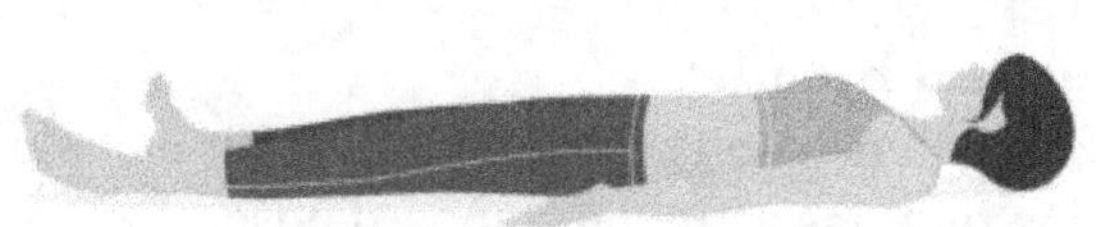

Lie Down

- Lie flat on your back on a comfortable surface, like a yoga mat.

Position Your Legs

- Separate your legs slightly, allowing your feet to fall open to either side.

Position Your Arms

- Place your arms alongside your body but slightly away from your torso. Turn your palms upward, letting your fingers naturally curl in.

Tuck Your Shoulders

- Tuck your shoulder blades under your back for support, similar to the movement in Bridge Pose but less intense.

Release Effort

- Once your limbs are positioned, release any effort in holding them in place. Let your body feel heavy and completely relaxed.

Natural Breathing

- Breathe naturally. If your mind wanders, simply return to your breath without forcing it.

Duration

- Stay in Savasana for at least five minutes. Ten minutes is ideal. If practicing at home, set an alarm to avoid checking the time.

Reawaken

- Begin to deepen your breath, then wiggle your fingers and toes to slowly reawaken your body.

Full Body Stretch

- A full-body stretch from hands to feet requires overhead arm stretching.

Fetal Position

- Roll onto one side with your knees in your chest and your lower arm as a pillow. Hold this position and breathe.

Sitting Up

- Using your hands for support, gently bring yourself back up to a sitting position.

Key Points

- Focus on relaxing each part of your body, one at a time.
- Let your breath come in and out of your body as it normally would.
- Stay conscious and alert, avoiding the temptation to fall asleep.

Variation:

Support the Head and Knees
- Place a folded blanket or bolster under your head and neck for support. Use a rolled blanket under your knees to relieve lower back tension.

Positioning
- Follow the same steps as the standard Corpse Pose, with the added supports in place.

Relax and Breathe
- Allow your body to relax fully with the added support, and follow the natural breathing instructions as in the standard pose.

Front Corpse Pose (Advasana)

Lie Down on Your Stomach
- Start by lying flat on your stomach with your legs extended straight behind you.
- Place your arms alongside your body with your palms facing up.

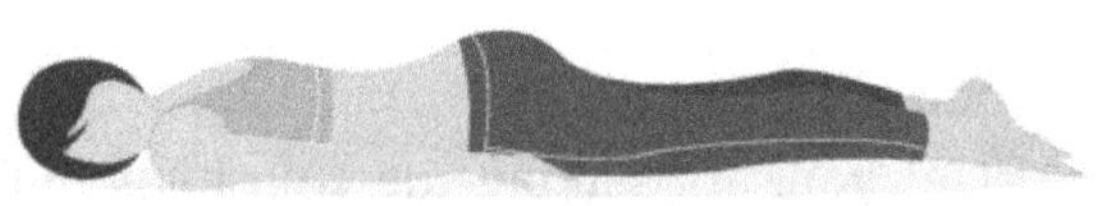

Extend and Relax
- Allow your legs to be hip-width apart or together, whichever is more comfortable.
- Let your toes point outwards naturally.

Extend Your Arms
- Extend your arms above your head, keeping them straight and shoulder-width apart.
- Rest your forehead on the floor.

Relax and Breathe
- Close your eyes and begin to relax each part of your body, starting from your toes and moving up to your head.
- Breathe deeply and slowly, allowing your body to sink into the floor with each exhale.

Hold the Pose
- Stay in the pose for 3 to 5 minutes, maintaining steady and deep breathing.
- Focus on releasing any tension in your body with each exhale.

Return to Starting Position
- To come out of the pose, gently bring your arms back to your sides.
- Slowly lift your head and chest off the floor, coming back to a neutral position.

Restorative yoga posture Supta Baddha Konasana, or Reclined Bound Angle Pose, offers deep relaxation and renewal. This pose helps release tension in the chest, abdomen, groins, and legs while also calming the mind and slowing the breath. It's particularly beneficial for relieving menstrual cramps, PMS, and digestive issues, making it one of the few yoga poses recommended after eating. Whether you need to relax before sleep or recharge during the day, this pose offers a gentle yet effective way to ground and connect with your body.

Begin in Baddha Konasana

- Seated on the floor, extend your legs. Bend your knees, draw your heels toward your pelvis, and drop your knees open. Put your feet together.

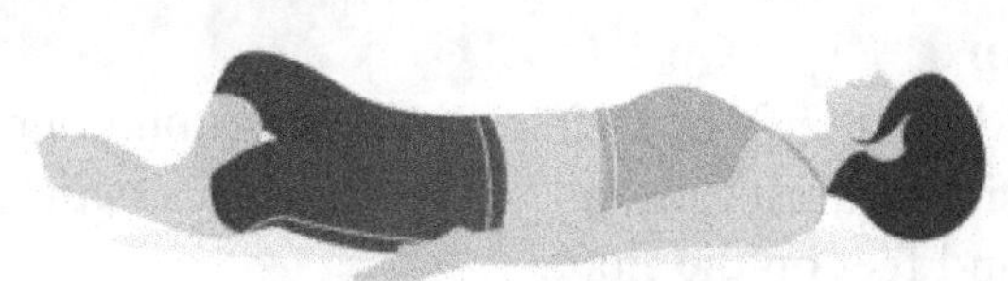

Lower to the Floo

- Breathe out and stoop down so your hands support your weight as you bring your upper body to the floor.
- Lean back on your forearms and spread your pelvis with your hands.
- Take a deep breath through your tailbone to relax your lower back and upper buttocks.
- Lower your body to the floor, and if necessary, use a bolster or blanket roll to prop up your head and neck.

Adjust Your Thighs

- By firmly grasping your upper thighs, you may turn your inner thighs outward while pressing your outer thighs away from your body.
- Run your hands over your outer thighs from hips to knees to expand and slide them away from your hips.
- As you imagine your inner groins sinking into your pelvis, slide your hands down your inner thighs, from the knees to the groins.

Position Your Arms

- Palms up, lay your arms on the floor 45 degrees from your torso.

Relax and Breathe

- Maintain your groins deep in your pelvis while imagining your knees rising up to the ceiling.
- As your groins drop toward the floor, your knees will follow.
- Start with one minute in this stance and work up to five to 10 minutes.

To Come Out

- Use your hands to press your thighs together.
- Push yourself off the floor with your head trailing your torso.

Key Points

- Use props like blankets or bolsters under your head and lower back if needed for comfort and proper alignment.
- Rotate your inner thighs externally and imagine your knees floating upward to prevent strain and deepen the groin stretch.
- Focus on deep, slow breaths to enhance relaxation and facilitate the release of tension in your muscles.

It is well-known that the calming effects of the yoga posture known as Legs Up the Wall Pose (also called Viparita Karani) can be felt both physically and mentally. Despite its simplicity, this pose offers profound benefits, including improved circulation, reduced swelling, and stress relief. It is an excellent choice for unwinding after a long day or incorporating it into your bedtime routine. By allowing your legs to rest against a wall, Viparita Karani helps reverse the downward flow of energy and blood, promoting relaxation and healing.

Setup

- Sit on the floor facing a wall. Position your side against the wall with your knees bent and feet on the floor.

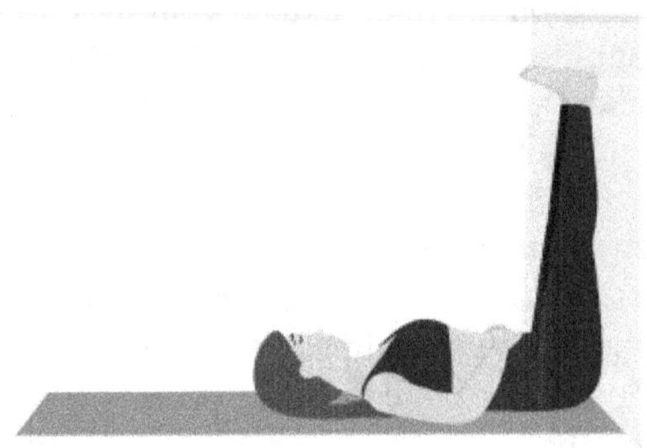

Transition

- As you lie on your side, bring your head and shoulders down to the floor. Then, as you're on your back, swing your legs up the wall. Get into a posture where your tailbone is almost touching the wall, but not quite touching.

Position Your Legs

- Raise your legs parallel to the wall, making sure they are hip-width apart or at a comfortable distance for you.

Relax Your Arms

- Put your arms at your sides, palms up. Arms and shoulders, relax.

Settle In

- Your legs will thank you when you let them relax against the wall. As you let your thighbones sink into your hip joints, you should also feel your spine lengthen. Relax into the position and take a few deep breaths.

Duration

- Breathe deeply and relax in the pose for 10 minutes.

Exit the Pose

- Roll to one side and bend your knees to exit. Wait a few breaths before carefully pushing yourself up to a seated position with your arms.

Key Points

- Allow your legs to rest fully against the wall and release all effort.
- Breathe deeply and steadily to enhance relaxation and stress relief.
- Ensure your spine feels long and supported, adjusting your position as needed for comfort.

Variation:

Setup with Props
- Place a folded blanket or bolster under your hips for added support.

Positioning
- Follow the same steps as the standard Legs Up the Wall Pose, with your hips elevated on the support.

Relax and Breathe
- Allow your body to settle into the pose, maintaining deep, steady breaths and enjoying the additional support from the props.

Lotus Pose, or Padmasana, is a classic seated posture in yoga that symbolizes tranquility, enlightenment, and the opening of the heart. This pose is deeply rooted in meditation practices and is often used for pranayama (breath control) and dhyana (meditation). Padmasana helps to calm the mind, strengthen the spine, and improve posture, making it an essential pose for those seeking to deepen their meditation practice and enhance their overall sense of well-being.

Starting Position

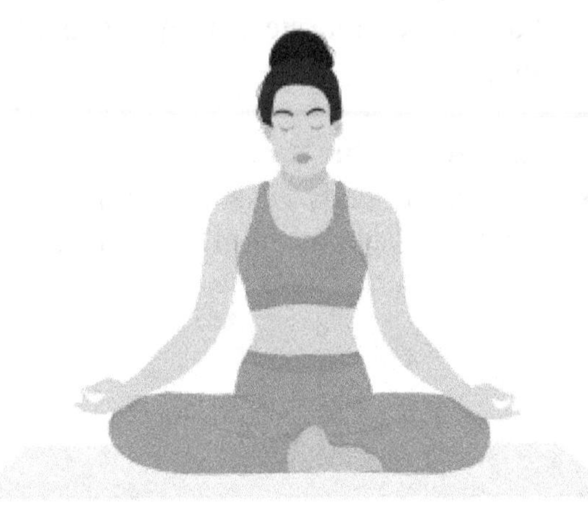

- Sit on your yoga mat with your legs extended straight in front of you (Dandasana/Staff Pose).
- Keep your spine straight and shoulders relaxed.

Position Your Right Foot

- Bend your right knee and bring your right foot up, placing it on your left thigh. The sole of your right foot should face upward, and the heel should be close to your abdomen.

Position Your Left Foot

- Bend your left knee and bring your left foot up, placing it on your right thigh. The sole of your left foot should also face upward, and the heel should be close to your abdomen.
- Ensure that both knees are touching the floor or are as close to the floor as possible.

Adjust Your Hips and Knees

- Use your hands to adjust your knees and thighs, ensuring that they are comfortable and well-supported.
- If necessary, place a cushion or blanket under your hips to elevate your pelvis and reduce strain on your knees.

Position Your Hands

- Rest your hands on your knees with your palms facing upward.
- You can also place your hands in a mudra (gesture) of your choice, such as Jnana Mudra (index finger and thumb touching) or Chin Mudra (palms facing down).

Lengthen Your Spine

- Sit up tall, lengthening through the crown of your head.
- Draw your shoulders back and down, away from your ears.

Focus on Your Breath

- Close your eyes and take several deep, calming breaths.
- Focus on maintaining a steady and relaxed breath throughout your practice.

Hold the Pose

- Stay in Lotus Pose for as long as comfortable, starting with a few minutes and gradually increasing the duration as your flexibility and comfort improve.

Key Points
- Ensure knees are close to the floor and the spine is lengthened. Use props if needed.
- Maintain a steady, relaxed breath to calm the mind.
- Gradually work on flexibility and comfort; avoid forcing the legs.

Appendix

Scan the QR Code and get your bonus.

Welcome to your 28-Day Yoga Journey, a transformative program designed to bring balance, flexibility, and strength to your body and mind. This plan is crafted to fit seamlessly into your daily routine, with each session lasting between 10 to 15 minutes. Whether you are a beginner or an experienced yogi, this program offers a diverse range of poses that will keep you engaged, challenged, and rejuvenated.

Why 28 Days? A 28-day commitment is perfect for creating and solidifying new habits. Over the next four weeks, you'll explore various yoga poses that target different parts of your body, ensuring a comprehensive and holistic approach to your practice. Each day brings a unique combination of poses designed to progressively build your flexibility, strength, and inner peace.

What to Expect

- **Daily Variety:** Each day offers a different set of poses, ensuring that you experience a wide range of yoga styles and benefits.
- **Balanced Practice:** The program includes poses that focus on the spine and core, shoulders and neck, legs and hips, full body flexibility, and relaxation. This balance ensures that no area of your body is neglected.
- **Mindful Breathing:** Each session emphasizes mindful breathing, helping you to stay present and deepen your practice.
- **Gradual Progression:** The sequence of poses is designed to gradually increase in complexity, allowing your body to adapt and grow stronger over time.

Getting Started: Find a quiet space where you can practice without distractions. Gather any props you might need, such as a yoga mat, blocks, or straps. Wear comfortable clothing that allows you to move freely. Remember, yoga is not about perfection; it's about making a connection with your body and mind.

Commit to Your Journey Embark on this 28-day journey with an open heart and a commitment to your well-being. By the end of the program, you will likely notice increased flexibility, strength, and a deeper sense of calm. Enjoy the process, listen to your body, and embrace each moment on your mat.

Day	Pose 1	Pose 2	Pose 3	Pose 4	Pose 5
1	Dandasana (Staff Pose)	Seated Forward Bend	Cat and Cow	Cobra Pose	Child's Pose
2	Tree Pose	Standing Lunge Stretch	Bound Angle Pose	Pigeon Pose	Reclined Big Toe Pose
3	Downward Facing Dog	Warrior I	Warrior II	Warrior III	Triangle Pose
4	Dolphin Pose	One-Legged Dolphin Pose	Sphinx Pose	Extended Puppy Pose	Happy Baby Pose
5	Boat Pose	Half Boat Pose	Bridge Pose	Supported Bridge Pose	Fish Pose
6	Spinal Twist	Seated Spinal Twist Variation	Cow Face Pose	Camel Pose	Rabbit Pose
7	Reclined Bound Angle Pose	Legs Up the Wall	Supine Figure Four	Cradle Baby Pose	Frog Pose
8	Hero Pose	Reclining Hero Pose	Lizard Pose	Modified Lizard Pose	Mermaid Pose
9	Goddess Pose	Goddess Twist Pose	Standing Forward Bend	Standing Forward Bend with Blocks	Warrior I
10	Warrior II	Warrior III	Triangle Pose	Triangle Pose with Brick	Extended Side Angle Pose
11	Extended Side Angle Pose with Brick	Half Moon Pose	Supported Half Moon Pose	Wheel Pose	Half Wheel Pose
12	Wheel Pose Using Chair	One-Legged Wheel Pose	Bow Pose	Half Bow Pose	Side Bow Pose
13	Corpse Pose	Support Corpse Pose	Front Corpse Pose	Reclined Bound Angle Pose	Legs Up the Wall
14	Dandasana (Staff Pose)	Seated Forward Bend with Block	Cat and Cow	Seated Cat-Cow	Cobra Pose with Bricks
15	Child's Pose with Arms Back	Spinal Twist	Boat Pose	Half Boat Pose	Bridge Pose
16	Supported Bridge Pose	Tiger Pose	Camel Pose	Camel Pose with a Chair	Fish Pose with a Chair
17	Fish Pose with Legs Crossed	Flying Fish Pose	Rabbit Pose	Locust Pose	Extended Locust Pose
18	Downward Facing Dog	Downward Dog Hand to Ankle	Three-Legged Downward Facing Dog	Downward Facing Dog with Block	Cow Face Pose
19	Cow Face Pose Variant Using a Strap	Thread the Needle Pose	Plow Pose	Wide-Legged Plow Pose	Extended Puppy Pose
20	Extended Puppy Pose with Blocks	Dolphin Pose	One-Legged Dolphin Pose	Tree Pose	Tree Pose Hand on the Wall
21	Standing Lunge Stretch	Kneeling Hip Flexor Stretch	Bound Angle Pose	Bound Angle Pose with Blocks	Pigeon Pose
22	Seated Pigeon Pose Using Chair	Pigeon Pose Using Block	One-Legged Pigeon Pose	King Pigeon Pose	Reclined Big Toe Pose
23	Reclined Big Toe Pose with a Strap	Happy Baby Pose	Happy Baby Pose With One Leg	Cradle Baby Pose	Frog Pose
24	Garland Pose	Supine Figure Four	Hero Pose	Reclining Hero Pose	Extended Reclining Hero Pose
25	Lizard Pose	Modified Lizard Pose with Knee Down	Monkey Pose	Twisted Monkey Pose	Mermaid Pose
26	Goddess Pose	Goddess Twist Pose	Standing Forward Bend	Standing Forward Bend with Blocks	Warrior I
27	Warrior II	Warrior II with a Chair	Warrior III	Wall Warrior III with Wall	Triangle Pose
28	Triangle Pose with Brick	Extended Side Angle Pose	Extended Side Angle Pose with Brick	Half Moon Pose	Supported Half Moon Pose

As we reach the end of our journey, it's essential to reflect on the transformative power of these practices. Throughout this book, we've explored a variety of yoga poses and somatic exercises, each designed to enhance your flexibility, improve respiration, and alleviate discomfort, particularly in the back and hips. From foundational poses like Dandasana (Staff Pose) to the more challenging Ardha Chandrasana (Half Moon Pose) and the restorative benefits of Savasana (Corpse Pose), each movement serves a unique purpose in fostering a deeper connection between mind and body.

The diverse range of poses covered in this book offers a comprehensive toolkit for beginners, empowering you to address various physical and mental needs. Whether you're looking to increase your flexibility with poses like Paschimottanasana (Seated Forward Bend), open your hips with poses like Baddha Konasana (Bound Angle Pose), or simply find relaxation and stress relief with Viparita Karani (Legs Up the Wall), there's something for everyone. These exercises are not just about physical fitness; they're about cultivating a mindful practice that enhances your overall well-being.

As we discussed, somatic exercises are particularly beneficial during pregnancy, providing a safe and effective way to stay active and manage the unique physical challenges of each trimester. Our carefully curated pregnancy yoga plan ensures that expectant mothers can continue to practice safely, adapting poses to accommodate their growing bellies and changing needs.
The journey of somatic exercise is a lifelong one, filled with continuous learning and self-discovery. It's about listening to your body, understanding its signals, and responding with compassion and care. Remember, the goal is not to achieve a perfect pose but to find ease and balance within each movement. As you progress, you'll find that the benefits extend beyond the mat, positively influencing your daily life and overall health.

Incorporating these exercises into your routine will help you build a strong foundation for a healthier, more mindful lifestyle. Continue to explore, adapt, and embrace the principles of somatic exercise, and you'll discover a profound sense of harmony between your body and mind.
Thank you for embarking on this journey with us. May your practice bring you peace, strength, and joy, now and always. Namaste.